MW01065127

You Had Me in Stitches
book that illustrates th
joy to be our strength in troubled times.
—Christina Federline

You Had Me in Stiches is an entertaining, realistic look at life with cancer and all the facets it entails. It helps you realize how much you must depend on a higher power (God) to get through this life with joy and expectancy. Mary was an inspiration during my own bout with cancer and I am truly blessed to call her "friend."
—Diane Hawkins

An informative journey through the eyes of one woman experiencing physical and emotional reactions to cancer. Follow her joyful approach to navigating the medical system and her courageous survival tactics. This is a great faith builder.
—Carol Means

You Had Me in Stitches

You Had Me in Stitches

A Breast Cancer Survivor Story

Mary Delacerda

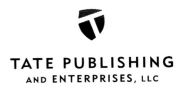

TATE PUBLISHING
AND ENTERPRISES, LLC

Published by Tate Publishing & Enterprises, LLC
127 E. Trade Center Terrace | Mustang, Oklahoma 73064 USA
1.888.361.9473 | www.tatepublishing.com

Tate Publishing is committed to excellence in the publishing industry. The company reflects the philosophy established by the founders, based on Psalm 68:11,
"The Lord gave the word and great was the company of those who published it."

Book design copyright © 2012 by Tate Publishing, LLC. All rights reserved.
Cover design by Blake Brasor
Interior design by Sarah Kirchen
Photo by The Sarah Image Photography

Published in the United States of America

ISBN: 978-1-61862-231-0
1. Biography & Autobiography / Personal Memoirs
2. Health & Fitness / Diseases / Cancer
12.03.20

This book is dedicated to my husband, Joe Delacerda.

Thank you for how you took care of me on the good days and on the bad days. For how you helped me with every treatment, every surgery, and every procedure from the beginning of my cancer diagnosis to the end of my healing process.

God gave me you!

I love you!
—Mary

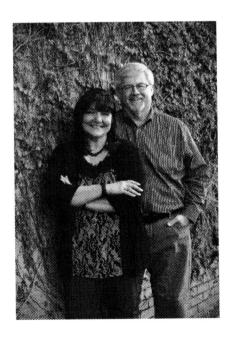

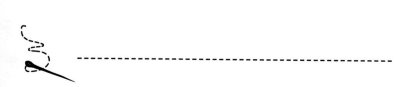

In loving memory of

William Emil Baab, Jr.

Better known as "Bud"

Or as we called him growing up "Buddy"

On January 10th, 2011

You entered Heaven

It was then I was encouraged to finish my book
and share my story

Your life exemplified your favorite quote…

Gaze at Christ; glance at everything else!

I miss you Bud!

Love you deeply,
—Mary

One verse—one very important verse:

> Consider it pure joy, my brothers, whenever you face trials of many kinds, because you know that the testing of your faith develops perseverance.

James 1:2-3 (NIV)

Acknowledgments

There are so many people I want to thank who really helped me along the way.

First of all, thank you to my Lord and Savior for how you sustained me and your Word encouraged me every single step of the way. Thank you for giving me a verse day one that would see me through this journey and teach me the true meaning of joy. Thank you for loving me so unconditionally. Thank you for knowing my needs before I knew them myself and meeting them through the people within my life. And most importantly, thank you for my relationship with you; for dying on that cross for my sins so that because of my belief in you, I have everlasting life.

Thank you to my husband who was there for every single need I had, and I mean the good, the bad, and, yes, the ugly. Thank you for praying with me and for me every day. I don't remember you ever complaining about a thing—not one single time. Thank you for listening. You did a lot of that! Thank you for giving me such security in your love for me during a time that could have been so insecure for me. You truly lived out our vows—in sickness and in health. Thank you!

Thank you to my children who made me laugh when I didn't feel like laughing. Thank you for the sacrifices each of you made for the past five years of your lives. Thank you for going to the store, cleaning the house, and doing the wash. Thank you for missing school to take care of your mom (this one I know you didn't mind). Thank you for understanding my absence at some of your school events when I was down after surgery. Thank you for allowing me to have a warped sense of humor sometimes and laughing with me. Thank you all.

Thank you to my extended family who helped take me to the doctor, took me out to lunch when I was unable to drive but needed to get out of the house, and just came and sat with me to keep me company.

Thank you to my friends and church family who provided cards, food, and flowers to cheer me up. Thank you for your encouragement and for continually praying for me.

Thank you to my doctors and nurses who cared for me along the way. There are many of you and you don't even realize how much you meant to me. Thank you for your kind words when I had questions. Thank you for your gentle touch when I was hurting after a surgery or procedure. Thank you for your constant care from the moment I walked into the hospital until I went home.

And last but not least, thank you to other cancer patients who just knew when I needed a hug. Thank you for not being afraid to show me your scars so I would understand what I should expect after surgery. Thank you for not being afraid or embarrassed to share your stories so I would feel normal. Thank you for recognizing me as one of you.

Each of you played a significant role in my life for the past five years. You may not realize it, but God strategically placed you there to help me through my journey. Thank you.

Table of Contents

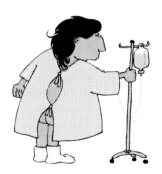

Introduction

A couple of years ago I wrote a book about my parents and the cancer that took both of their lives. First it came into my mom's life when she was forty-four years old and then my dad was diagnosed soon after he turned sixty-nine. I never thought that cancer would be part of either of their lives, nor did I think they would both die from it. But God used their experiences to help me with my eventual bout with cancer. Yes, at the age of forty-four, I too was diagnosed with cancer—breast cancer.

As I look back over the past nineteen years, I see how God has changed me and prepared me for my own personal journey with cancer.

Incredibly, I had an amazing peace through it all, and I didn't have cancer just once but twice. I have spent the past seven years in awe of how God has walked me through it all and with a considerable amount of joy. Yes, I have had great joy in spite of it all. Early on, God gave me a verse from his Word to hold on to. It is from the book of James.

> Consider it pure joy my brothers, whenever you face trials of many kinds, because you know that the testing of your faith develops perseverance.
>
> James 1:2-3 (NIV)

Throughout my journey, God consistently brought me back to this verse over and over again.

I serve an awesome God and Savior, and I thank him for sustaining my life so I could share my journey with you.

So, let's consider it pure joy together...

My Family

Before I share my cancer story with you, I wanted to tell you a little about my family.

I was born in New Brunswick, New Jersey. I only lived there for a couple of years before my dad moved us to San Angelo, Texas. We lived there for several years, and then we moved to Arlington, Texas. When I was eight or nine, we moved to Tulsa, Oklahoma, which is where I have lived ever since. My husband and I reside in Jenks, Oklahoma, which is a suburb of Tulsa.

I come from a family of eight; my parents and six children. I am the third child with two older brothers, two younger brothers and one younger sister.

I went to Jenks Public Schools starting in the fourth grade until I graduated in May of 1977. I was a good student and cheered for Jenks all through my high school years. I then went on to Oklahoma State University where I graduated with a bachelor's degree in psychology in May of 1981.

I married my boyfriend (also from Jenks) of four years in January of 1981. We lived in the married student housing in Stillwater for the first year of his graduate program and moved back to Tulsa while he commuted to school the last year. We then bought a house in Glenpool and lived there until our first son was two years old. We moved to Jenks at that point and have lived there ever since.

We have now been married for thirty years and have raised three children—two boys and one girl. We also have one grandson who is ten-years-old.

We have also been active members of Jenks First Baptist Church since 1983. I taught youth Sunday school for about 10 years. I am now involved in the women's ministry there, and I also help lead in the Women's Bible Studies.

I enjoy time with my husband, my children, and my grandson. In my spare time I love to walk, bake, and, of course, write. God is good!

What Did You Say?

The year was 2004. It was the Monday morning of spring break, and I was waiting on a call from my doctor who took a biopsy the Friday before. She wanted to make sure the specks they saw on my mammogram were nothing to be concerned about. I wasn't too concerned since she said she was 95 percent sure it was nothing—pretty good odds.

I had been told the Friday before to expect a call around noon when things had calmed down from the morning. So, I was hard at my Monday morning cleaning. Weekends were always busy and I never had time to clean until the weekend was over. Three children and a grandchild was enough to keep me busy. Around 9:15 in the morning, the phone rang and sure enough, it was my doctor.

"Good morning, Mary," she said in a very sweet voice. She seemed to carry on for quite a while with her pleasantries. I liked her a lot because she seemed to be such a compassionate female doctor; she also seemed to truly know what to say or not say to me, the patient. "Your results are in," she said. "You have what is called ductal carcinoma in sutu." In that very moment, I couldn't believe I had just heard the word *carcinoma.* I had heard that word before; it meant cancer. *Cancer, as in cancer like my mom's cancer,* was all I could think. Absolutely nothing came out of my mouth for several seconds and then I blurted out, "What did you say?" She very gently repeated the medical title for it and kept talking. From that point on, what she said, I couldn't tell; not one word was sinking in. All I could do was sit there and try to comprehend that I had just been told I had cancer. Finally, I remember hearing her say, "If you have any questions, call me, and please make an appointment with a surgeon as soon as possible."

When I hung up the phone, I realized that since I hadn't heard a thing she said, I would have to call her back and ask her to repeat herself. So I did. She was so very nice about it; she said that happens all the time because very few people hear beyond that word—*cancer.*

When It Rains: It Pours

It was the beginning of 2004, and I decided it was time to take care of those female appointments. I had not been feeling great (I was having a lot of cramping throughout the month), so I made an appointment with my gynecologist.

My gynecologist is a great doctor. He delivered all three of my children and had helped counsel me through some difficulties throughout the past fifteen years of my life. I considered him a friend and fully trusted him. Since I had been cramping a lot for the past several months, I knew something was not right. After a check-up, he felt it would be necessary to do a D&C, a Dilation and Curettage, to see what the problem was. This procedure enabled my doctor to actually see the problem and then know what steps were necessary to stop my cramping.

I was so nervous about this procedure. *Oh my goodness, they will have to put me to sleep*, I thought. I wasn't very thrilled about that. The only other time I had been put to sleep was when my second son was born, and that was done during his delivery due to some complications.

The procedure was to be done two weeks later. That was a long two weeks of me wondering, "Will I wake up when it's over?" Or worse, "Will I wake up in the middle of the procedure?" I look back at it and just laugh to think that I was so nervous about such a basic procedure, but I was truly a nervous wreck thinking about it all the time. Little did I know that I would have twelve more surgeries in the next seven years that were huge compared to this one.

Finally, the day came for the procedure. I was so uptight and a bit shaky. My hands and feet were so cold. When they took me back to the operating room, I just remember lying on that table and thinking, "Okay, Lord, I am in your hands; it is up to you to help me get through this. Calm me Lord, just give me a scripture or two, right now."

Then, as clear as can be, the scripture from James 1:2-3 came to my mind. It says, "Consider it pure joy, my brothers, whenever you face trials of many kinds, because you know that the testing of your faith develops perseverance." I knew in that very moment that it was going to be the scripture that would help me through whatever road God chose for me; I just didn't realize how many joy moments were ahead of me on this journey.

Of course, I came through with flying colors. I woke up about an hour later and felt totally normal. I had heard that a D&C is pretty painless, and that is absolutely true. I was so glad it was done. Part of me was mad at myself for my lack of faith for the past couple of weeks. God took very good care of me throughout it all, and I knew he would. I should have trusted him more.

When my doctor came into my recovery room, his news was not good. He said I had a severe case of endometriosis, and I needed a complete hysterectomy. Because I'd had c-sections with all three of my children, he felt the best way to do this surgery was abdominally. *Darn, that means I have to go back to sleep again and be cut on this time.* I don't like having my stomach cut on; it hurts. It hurts a lot! This would be the fourth time for him to cut my stomach open. That seems just wrong. But, I couldn't argue with my doctor. He knew what was best, so we set it up for two weeks later.

Now here I go again. That was another long two weeks. Not only was I worrying about being put to sleep, but this time they would cut me open and I would hurt afterwards. I never thought of myself as anything less than healthy, and I wasn't enjoying this journey at all.

Two weeks finally went by, and there I was, sitting in my pre-op room again with my gown that allows people to peek at your backside. I wasn't quite as nervous about going to sleep this time. Actually, I welcomed it because of what they had to do. Lord knows, I wanted to be knocked out for that. It was to be a three hour surgery. That sounded so long to me, but at least I was the one asleep and not the one in the waiting room.

My husband was the recipient of that job. He wasn't very thrilled about all this either, but like me, he knew it was necessary. Of course, my children and some friends also came to help the time pass by. Thank goodness for family and friends; they are such a blessing.

Three hours passed, and my surgery was complete. When I awoke, I was overwhelmed with how I felt. I had never known such pain before; childbearing was a piece of cake compared to this. I was in recovery, and I just kept asking for more pain medicine; I cried a lot. My nurse was very nice but finally told me that, if she gave me anything else, I could die. I guess I wasn't handling my pain too well. I also had uncontrollable shakes, but was able to drift in and out of sleep, which seemed to help me a little.

I was in recovery for over two hours before they took me to my room. When I saw my husband, I just started crying. I guess my emotions just got the best of me, and seeing him just made me lose it.

I stayed in the hospital for two more days, and then my doctor sent me home—with my pain medicine, thank goodness. I watched the clock to take those pills. This was not a fun experience for me, and I chose to be as numb as possible. It seemed the only way for me to handle it.

After arriving home my husband brought in the mail. There it was—a letter from my doctor's office. As I read it, I couldn't believe my eyes. It said that there were some abnormalities on my mammogram—which I had 3 weeks earlier—that concerned them. They felt a biopsy should be done just to make sure it was nothing serious. Immediately I called and asked about the procedure. When I told the doctor at the mammogram office what I had just had done, she suggested that I wait a couple of weeks and come in when I felt better since I would have to lay on my stomach for this biopsy. "Are you kidding" I said. I couldn't wait a couple of weeks to know if everything was okay. I told her I would be in the next week with a pillow, and I would somehow manage to have that biopsy. So, I had a new goal—to get better quickly. I also figured it would be wise to take a couple of pain pills the morning of the biopsy so I wouldn't be so miserable.

Everything I have ever heard about biopsies was not good. Everyone I've ever talked to said they hurt like crazy, and they would never forget their biopsy. Great, it looked like I had so much to look forward to.

Again, I was waiting on time to pass for another procedure. *This is beginning to get old*, I thought. *I am 44 years old. Why am I having so many problems? Am I not healthy?*

The morning came for my biopsy; it was a Friday. I felt I had planned that well since my family would be home to help me if I was extra sore. I took two pain pills and off I went to the doctor. I had to wait quite a while; they were behind on the schedule that day. Waiting is not something I do very well, especially if I know pain will probably follow. Finally, it was my turn. The nurses chuckled at my pillow but praised me for coming in so quickly. It took me at least ten minutes to get on the table with my pillow. I was far from comfortable, but I did it. So, the biopsy began.

This is such a barbaric procedure. The doctor makes a small incision to reach the concerned area of the breast, a small medical tool is placed by the incision, and the doctor reaches in quickly and tears a piece of tissue out. They took eleven samples and put them in a petri dish, showing them to me as the procedure went on. They only gave me a little numbing medicine, and after the third sample, I had to let the doctor know I couldn't do another sample until they gave me more medicine. They put butterfly band-aids on me and said to take it easy for the day because I wouldn't feel too good. That was the understatement of the day. I bled right through my band-aids and my bra, and, of course, I was wearing a white blouse and bled through that too. I felt like I needed to hold that poor breast. It had just been so violated as far as I was concerned. No wonder everyone says biopsies are no fun. They are awful; just awful. I was in tears the whole way home. It hurt every time my husband went over even the smallest of bumps. I made it to the couch when I got home and took more medicine immediately. I just wanted to go to sleep and not think about it anymore.

It took me a couple of days to feel back to normal, but I healed and all I needed was that phone call on Monday to let me know everything was fine although I was told not to worry.

Here Comes the Joy

I have just hung up the phone from the doctor for the second time, and I realize there is so much to think about and do.

I asked my husband to call my dad and tell him about my diagnosis while I took a quick shower. I knew my dad well enough to know he would be at my house within ten minutes of learning I had cancer.

Plus, the shower was my opportunity to just think without anyone interrupting me. As I stood in the shower, it was almost like I could hear him out loud. It was the Lord; I knew it as sure as I know anything. He said, "Child of mine, let it go and give it to me. This is not in your control, it is in mine. Let it go." I felt this huge release and a joy in knowing I didn't have to do this by myself. It was not for me to do. It was God's problem; not mine. I had total peace like I have never known it before. As I was getting dressed (because, yes, my dad was in the kitchen already), I dressed myself with a lot more than my clothing; I was dressed with the armor of God. I knew it from that very moment.

As I walked out of the bedroom, I had no tears. I didn't need them. I was able to smile, hug my dad, and share with him my thoughts without any trouble.

I did have one amazing blunder while talking to my dad. Of course he was extremely concerned like any parent would be. As we were talking, he said to me, "I will help you through this any way I can." My husband and I had just watched our son go through a very rough time and without thinking I said to Dad, "I am fine, Dad. As long as God doesn't put another hardship in my son's life, I can handle whatever is in mine. I just can't bear to watch my child suffer." It was quiet for a moment or two when Dad responded, "Remember, *you* are my child." My dad had just learned his child had cancer. It didn't matter if I was ten or fifty. I was still his child. As we talked, we both agreed that it was God who would truly get us through this time.

I gave my dad a hug and sent him home so my husband and I could get to work learning more about the specific cancer I had and finding a surgeon.

I felt like someone just put me out in the dark without a flashlight and told me to find my way home. But that was okay. I knew that God was my flashlight and he would help me figure out what road to take through this journey.

Surgeon Number One—NOT!

After talking to many people, including those with access to and knowledge of the medical field, I was convinced of the group of doctors I wanted to use. When I called to make an appointment, I was fortunate that they had an opening for the very same week on a Thursday. In the meantime, I searched the internet and the local library for absolutely everything I could read or learn about my cancer. There was just so much to learn, and I couldn't read enough about it. It gave me a sense of power to know more about what my body was dealing with and the different ways I could treat it.

My boys were rather appalled at how many books on breasts were lying around the house suddenly. We joked about that frequently.

Thursday arrived before I knew it, and I was very ready to meet my doctor. The office was very nice and looked professional, and I had a good feeling about it. Once back in the room, the doctor came in. I was quite surprised to see that he didn't look but maybe twenty-two-years-old. His approach was different from what I was expecting. I guess I was expecting him to be very aggressive in his thinking since my mom had died of breast cancer a couple years ago. Instead, he used new-age thinking, as far as I was concerned. He suggested we do a lumpectomy and radiation, all to save the breast. Well, sure that would be nice, but I would rather save my life than my breast. Then he said he would consider doing several lumpectomies before doing a mastectomy.

A lumpectomy is a procedure where the doctor removes tissue about the size of an egg from the concerned area. If several lumpectomies are done on one breast, it would leave that breast ugly and poorly shaped. Plus, who gets cancer several times and hasn't figured out it is time to do something more serious than another lumpectomy? My husband and I considered this a joy moment just because it seemed so absurd to us.

In our family (my husband and my children) we tend to find and even look for laughter in everything. It just helps us as we travel a difficult journey. So, yes, my husband and I were laughing.

Because I didn't have the nerve to say what I was thinking, I agreed to the surgery and set it up for the next week. I just didn't know what to say, and I didn't want to hurt the doctor's feelings.

The moment we were out of that office, I looked my husband straight in the face and said "I am not going back there—ever. Not to that doctor." So, we called and canceled that surgery.

Once again, we were back to finding a surgeon.

Surgeon Number Two—Practice Makes Perfect

So, we did more research and again, found a doctor we thought would be perfect for me.

This time, it wasn't so easy to get in. I had to wait over two weeks just to see him. Maybe that was a good thing. If he was so busy, that was probably because everyone else wanted to see him too.

That was a long two-plus weeks waiting to see him. Every day I woke up and I knew I had this cancer in me just growing more and more until I could get it out. That is just an awful feeling because a part of my body had turned on me, and it is going to make the rest of my body sick if I didn't do something about it. I just felt such an urgency to address my cancer.

The day finally arrived for me to see the second surgeon. I really liked his nurse; she was very kind and gentle—the perfect nurse for my situation. When the doctor came in he was much older than the first surgeon I met. I liked that. As far as I was concerned, age meant wisdom. He asked a lot of questions about my family history and decided he wanted to do a heredity test on me before he decided what surgery was best. I immediately liked him. He was thorough—like me.

The heredity test took three weeks though, and that meant three more weeks of that cancer in me. But, I knew it was the right thing to do. The test was easy; lots of questions and then they simply took some blood. The three weeks were a long, hard wait. They went by very slowly. My husband didn't like the wait; my kids didn't either. Even my dad didn't like those three weeks. It was just a lot of waiting. But as any Christian knows, it is in the waiting for things in our life that God grows us in our walk with him. So, yes, I was also growing closer to God day by day.

Finally, the three weeks were up and the doctor called. The entire test showed that I was negative for being a hereditary carrier of cancer. That was such good news. Now my doctor was comfortable with doing a lumpectomy; only because of those results. I would then need to follow up with eight weeks of radiation, but I was okay with that. I just wanted to feel like I was doing the right surgery for the cancer I had.

So, finally, we were able to schedule my surgery for the next week. Again, I would get on that operating table. Might I mention that it was the third time in a year that I would be having surgery? Is this becoming a joke? I didn't even need a new pre-op appointment, because my pre-op was still good from my last surgery. Yes, I would call this a *joy* moment, even if it is just enough to make me smile or giggle to myself a little.

Which Breast?
The One with the
Wire Hanging Out!

In every procedure I have been through over the years there is always humor. Little did I know that this next surgery would be the one that we look back at and laugh the most.

The day of the lumpectomy had finally arrived. I was truly ready for this surgery. Going to sleep no longer scared me since I had done it twice before and very recently at that.

Prior to coming to the hospital I was told to go by the office where they performed the mammogram so they could wire me. I wasn't sure what that meant, but I just followed their instructions. They also told me to wear a loose fitting blouse for comfort. As I arrived at the office, they did not keep me waiting since they knew I had a scheduled surgery. They took me right in. Now keep in mind, I could not eat or drink the night before and I was probably a little nervous too. As they took me back and explained this procedure, I began to stress. They did a mammogram and kept my breast in the machine as they stuck the wire in the breast to the exact location of the cancer. This is done with no pain medicine or numbing at all.

So, there I was, standing in another one of those lovely gowns and I was secured (or at least my breast was) in the mammogram machine. The doctor told me they will penetrate the breast about an inch at a time. Unfortunately my cancer was about five inches within the breast. That meant they would have to do this in five steps. I did appreciate her honesty though; she said it would hurt.

So, it was time to get started. She let me know that they were getting ready to start putting in the wire. Oh my goodness—*ouch*! I was able to do the first three penetrations okay, but then I started to get very faint. I told them and they brought me a chair that I could sit in for a few minutes. They even adjusted the mammogram machine so it could sit down with me. Here I am sitting down with my hospital gown, my breast in that machine, and a wire hanging out of it. If I didn't hurt so much, maybe I could have laughed, but nothing seemed funny at the moment.

Finally after about ten minutes I felt a little better. I needed to let them get the final two penetrations done so I could get over to the hospital for my surgery. I just gritted my teeth and said, "Let's get this over with." After they got the wire in far enough, they had me put my blouse back on. They coiled up all the extra wire under my arm and said to be very careful so it stays exactly in place. That is very important for the surgeon during the surgery.

Once out of the office, I met my husband in the waiting room, and we left to go to the hospital. He could tell I was hurting and uncomfortable to say the least. I was walking around with a wire hanging out of the side of my left breast. Now that's just wrong!

We arrived at the hospital and went right to registration. They put me in a room and my husband and I actually laughed at the entire process. Several nurses came in to ask their questions. Of course, each one wanted me to remind them which breast it was that was being operated on that day. At one point, my husband just couldn't help himself anymore. He responded, "It would be the one with the wire hanging out of it." Let's just say, *joy, joy, joy* for this moment. We just found the whole thing so darn funny the more we thought about it. We were actually laughing to the point of tears. Though not everyone has a warped sense of humor like my husband and I do, surely this time would be funny to anyone who actually saw that wire!

Finally, it was time to go back to surgery. If nothing else, I was ready to be without that wire hanging out of my breast. The surgery only took about an hour and I was sent to recovery. It was an out-patient procedure, so I knew I didn't have to stay in the hospital which was nice. When I woke up, my pain was manageable. I was tender on that breast, but this was nothing like my hysterectomy. My doctor sent me home to heal and told me he would call with the results of the pathology report. That would tell them if they felt they got it all.

One other thing that was too funny (another *joy* moment) was that the nurse wrote 'yes' on the breast I told her they were operating on. Then when the doctor came in to ask a few questions, he too wrote yes on that breast. After the surgery was over, I noticed I had a third yes written on that breast (probably done after I had been put to sleep). Needless to say, I guess they all wanted to make sure they operated on the correct one—too funny. I went home with "yes, yes, yes" on that breast!

It only takes a couple of days to recover from a lumpectomy. The only noticeable difference is a small incision on the side of my breast and a hollow feeling where they took the cancer out.

I was so glad that it was over with. I had already been told that thirty-three rounds of radiation are standard, so I was ready to move forward and prepare for the next battle of this journey.

About a week later the doctor called to tell me they got all the cancer—praise God! He felt we got it early enough that it would not come back. It was time now to start my radiation.

Radiation did not scare me at all. I was so grateful I didn't have to have chemotherapy. The only horror stories I had actually heard with radiation was usually by the end of it you could be burned in the radiated area.

So, I went to my initial appointment for the radiation. That day, all they did was tattoo me. They put two permanent tattoos (they look like beauty marks) on each side of that breast. This helps as they are positioning me for my specific radiation.

Of course, later that day, when my husband came home, I couldn't help but have a little fun with it and let him know his wife had two tattoos now. *Joy!* I firmly believe it is not by chance that there was humor in all of this. Not only did God allow that humor but he did so that we would know that laughing was good through it all. Little did we know there was much more laughter to come.

Radiation was done every day, for five days a week until my cycle was complete. My cycle was to last thirty-three days. The thing I liked about my cycle was it would be done by Friday, July 1 and we planned to celebrate it as my freedom from cancer over the July Fourth weekend. So, I was committed to getting it done without any interruptions. My scheduled time was eight in the morning every day. I would grow to dislike the time I chose, but at least it only took fifteen minutes and I was done. It actually took me longer to get there and back than to get the radiation.

So the first day for radiation arrived and I walked in and was caught a little off guard because it was me and all older women and men. That upset me more than I expected. It just made me think, *Why am I here, I am too young for this.*

When my turn came, I went back into a big, cold room. It was such an easy process. They lay you in a position so they can radiate the specific area. You have to lie completely still. They leave the room. The radiation machine turns on. It takes a total of five minutes. You get dressed and you are done. It's that simple—a piece of cake. *I can do this,* I thought.

The first couple of weeks went by quickly, but I did start to realize I picked a time that is too early. Summer had started, and the only reason I was getting out of the house that early was to go to radiation. I didn't have to get out early to take my children to school, so why did I schedule such early radiation treatments? If nothing else, it was done for the day so I could go home and enjoy summertime with my children.

I did notice there was one other young woman. Actually, she was younger than me by probably ten years. She always wore long sleeves, and I could tell she had had a mastectomy and no reconstruction. She would go in right before me, so I saw here every day.

As the weeks went by, I laughed at my routine. I would go a little early to ensure I didn't miss my time. I found myself gravitating to the puzzle table (set up for cancer patients to help preoccupy us while waiting for our treatment) with the older women. I made friends with them and heard their stories. I grew close to them and looked forward to seeing them each day. We bonded. We were all in this together. The young woman before me never came early and we never chatted, but she was always pleasant and smiled as she left.

One week, on a Friday, the machine was down. We all waited for an hour at least, and the technician came out saying they were not sure what time it would be up and running. I was so frustrated. I was committed to completing my radiation on time, so I decided to wait no matter how long it took to fix the machine. If nothing else, I was able to work on the puzzle a lot that day.

After about three hours the machine was finally up and running. Most of the other cancer patients left out of frustration, but not me. I was ready for my radiation. It took just a couple of minutes to complete, and I was on my way.

I had two weeks left at this point, and I was really anxious to be done. Finally, the last day of radiation arrived. It was also the last day for the other young woman with cancer. As I arrived that day, I was in for a bit of a shock. She had just completed her last treatment and walked out with such a smile. She was not covered up this time. She was celebrating her last treatment with not only a smile, but the decision not to cover up her wounds. She was so badly burnt. I had burned a little, but nothing like her. I was so shocked by what I saw, but how it ministered to me. I was just so blessed by how carefree she looked, and yet I knew she had suffered a lot in her last few weeks of radiation. I think it was God's way of showing me my situation could have been worse. I went home that day praying for her and continued to pray for her for weeks following. God laid her on my heart frequently during those weeks which helped remind me to pray for her.

I completed my last radiation treatment that day and went home to a great Fourth of July celebration. We celebrated my freedom from cancer, my freedom from treatment, and my healing.

Even though I knew I would go to checkups every three months, I was so excited to know cancer was no longer in my life.

It took me no time at all to feel back to normal and live my normal day to day life. I did not dwell on my cancer coming back. I truly didn't think about. I just trusted God.

Check-up Time—
That is, Check-up
Number Two

I actually had two types of checkups at this point of my recovery. First of all, I went in every three months to my breast surgeon just for routine checkups. He was very thorough and checked me closely. At this point, I did not find it embarrassing anymore because I just wanted his professional opinion for my peace of mind. Normally, I was such a shy and reserved patient about anything female related, but after all I had been through, I guess I felt differently about these checkups now.

The second checkups were my mammograms, of course. I was now having them every six months. My first six-month checkup was fine. No concerns at all. When my surgeon had done my lumpectomy, he left a tiny piece of metal in the location of where the cancer was so while they did my mammogram they would check that area extra close. I felt very good about that. I appreciated how thorough my doctor was with me.

During my second six-month checkup, things did not go as well. After they did the initial mammogram, the technician left me in the room for quite a long time.

I just started to get this funny feeling. I even called my husband while I was waiting in the room in my gown and told him I was a little concerned. I even said to him that if the technician walked in with the doctor, I knew that was not a good sign. Right as I said that, sure enough, they both came back into the room. I quickly hung up with my husband. Sure enough, they had a little concern about that same area. The doctor said it might just be scar tissue, but that didn't make much sense to me. Why did it not show up at the first six-month check up? They wanted to do a biopsy. Oh boy, you know how I feel about biopsies!

Over the next few years I would hear many stories of people who felt their biopsy was the worst part of their cancer experience—I agreed. Fortunately, this time they wanted to put me to sleep for it. I was okay with that. How great is that? Being put to sleep doesn't scare me at all at this point. I now actually like it. I like that great feeling you have the few seconds before you are knocked out. We joke about it in our home. My kids think I am a little crazy. For example, my children think I purposely planned more surgery all so I can have anesthesia. Now if I had a choice of no more surgery verses one more surgery for the sake of the anesthesia, I am sure I would pass on more surgery!

We scheduled the biopsy for later that week. It was a quick couple of days. That waiting time didn't bother me. I was comfortable with hospital procedures at this point. I knew all the questions they would ask and what to wear or not to wear the day of the procedure.

As they took me to the surgery room I remember thinking, *Will I have to take this sickness on again? Why won't this breast quit offending the rest of my body and stay well?*

The procedure went well. I woke up, again with manageable discomfort. Pain like this didn't bother me enough to complain or even take pain medicine, but I did fill my prescription just in case I felt bad later that evening. There are a few lessons I had already learned, and one was to not be off guard without any pain medicine late at night when the doctor's office was closed for the day, or worse, the weekend!

We were in the waiting mode for the results to come in. At that point I was comfortable in that mode.

The procedure had been done on a Friday so of course, my wait was over a weekend. It made for a long weekend. Monday did finally arrive. I waited all day for that call. All day.

Finally, about five-thirty in the evening the phone rang. My husband and our two younger children were at the table playing card games. I looked at the caller ID and said, "This is it. It's the doctor." I had already accepted the fact that it was probably cancer when I was in the doctor's office and the doctor said he had a concern. I just knew scar tissue did not make sense to me if it was not seen after that first check-up.

I answered the phone and sure enough my doctor was on the other end. He was very professional and got right to the point. I appreciated that after having waited all day. "I just received your test results Mary and wanted to call you immediately. Unfortunately, there is more cancer," he said. I repeated what he said so my family heard what I heard. I actually did not get upset as he said the cancer had returned to the exact same area. I listened as he discussed what process I should take from there and said thank you for letting me know this late in the day.

As I hung up the phone, I did a quick study of my husband, son, and daughter before saying a word. They all reacted so very differently.

My husband, I could tell, was upset but actually angry more than anything else. He was mad that it was back in my, or should I say our, lives. He knew that I would be very aggressive in the treatment the second time around. My mom died of cancer several years before, and I was going to do *everything* possible to preserve my life; even if it did mean a surgery that we were trying to avoid.

Then there was my second son. He was such a rock. I could feel his inner strength and courage as he sat across from me. He sat quiet, while my daughter was the first one to actually say anything.

My daughter is our youngest child and was three days away from starting her senior year. Her best friend had just moved out of state the week earlier, her brother (the one at the table with us) was leaving later that week for his freshman year of college and now, her mother was just told she had cancer…again. So, her senior year was getting off to a pretty rough start. She just looked at me with tears in her eyes and started to run up the stairs. I guess she just had to get out of the room so she could let her emotions go. As she was headed upstairs, I remember her saying something to the effect of, "Why you? You are such a good person. Why you?"

My husband started to leave the table as he needed some space also.

Somehow in the moment and with that sweet comment from my daughter, I vividly remember thinking, *Say something to lighten up the tension in this room — now!* I looked at my son, we both smiled, and I said, "Okay, I'll go talk to your Dad and you go upstairs and talk to your sister." My son and I just connected in that moment because we both knew the same thing: God was in control. We didn't even have to say a thing, we just knew it.

After a short while, I was able to contact my oldest son and let him know also. He is a very strong person as he had been through much in his life already. He was great on the phone in how he handled his responses. He was serving in the military and far away, so it helped to know that he was able to handle it that well. As everyone needed a little time to let it sink in, we knew it was time to get back to the business of getting rid of this cancer once again.

That night as we went to bed I reminded my husband that I would do *whatever* surgery was necessary to get rid of this cancer.

Cancer—Round 2

When my mom was diagnosed the second time with cancer, it scared me quite a bit. I was very frustrated that we were down that road again.

But, with my second diagnosis, I again had no fear. I did not lose any sleep either. Actually, I slept like a baby. Go figure! I now know that it was the presence of God in my life. I felt his presence constantly.

My husband went back to my surgeon with me. The surgeon said that during the biopsy he took a larger section of tissue and since we caught the second cancer so early, I was probably already cancer free. He also told me that they could not do radiation on the same location twice so there would be no radiation this time. *Okay, so what is next?* I thought.

I asked him what my percentages were of getting cancer back in that breast. He said it was about 40 percent. That was unbelievable! I looked my doctor straight in the eyes and said, "If I were your daughter," what would you tell her to do?" He hesitated and looked at me. I knew that by asking this question, I put him on the spot to give me his personal opinion and not just the typical doctor answer. He said, "If you were my daughter, I would probably encourage you to at least do a single mastectomy." That was all I needed to hear. I had some homework to do at this point, and I knew it.

As we left the doctor's office, I actually thought to myself, *Here I go again, surgery!*

Surgery—How Many Hours Long?

I had several options for surgery at this point.

- Single mastectomy

- Double mastectomy

- Single mastectomy with reconstruction

- Double mastectomy with reconstruction

Any of these would take care of the most important thing which was ensuring I would not get breast cancer back. I just had to decide which was right for me. And I would like to add that what was right for me might not be right for another woman.

Of course, my first thought was let's do what we have to do to ensure I don't have to deal with breast cancer again. Though my first thought was the single mastectomy, I knew my mom had had that and so disliked having a breast on one side and not the other. She even joked about having the one remaining breast put surgically in the middle so she wouldn't feel so lopsided. Maybe I got my warped sense of humor from my mom, as she had *joy* moments too. Unfortunately, I knew in the long run, I would not like the way it felt to have only one breast so I knocked that off the list of options.

My second option was to have a double mastectomy. I knew I didn't want to feel lopsided so the double mastectomy would be a better choice for me. Plus it would definitely lower my chances of getting breast cancer back again. This seemed like the better choice for me except for one minor detail. I didn't think I would feel complete with nothing there either. I was afraid I would not feel complete—like a whole woman—without breasts. We have a swimming pool and we like to vacation by the ocean, so I needed to feel and look like a woman. I didn't see myself as an insecure person, but if that option was available, I needed to check it out. So, I guess I could knock the second option off the list too.

Option number three—single mastectomy with reconstruction. Because I had radiation after my first cancer diagnosis, I have limited surgeries that I can do for my reconstruction. I cannot have implants done for my reconstruction because they cannot be done on a radiated area due to the possibility of an infection. Therefore, the only reconstruction options open to me were where they take tissue from one of two areas of my body and reconstruct my breast with it. Those two areas were either my stomach muscle or my back muscle. Either of these surgeries would be done by tunneling the tissue to the designated area. The downfall with having a single mastectomy and this reconstruction done is that if the other breast eventually becomes cancerous and I needed a mastectomy done on that side, I cannot do the reconstruction twice. It's a one time deal, so needless to say, this option is out also.

Option number four—the double mastectomy and reconstruction option. This, of course, is the hardest and biggest surgery. It requires removing more and replacing more tissue. It is also more painful and makes for a longer recovery.

After much thought and prayer, my husband and I knew it was the best option. My husband was less enthused than me because he was so concerned about the magnitude of the surgery. I decided the stomach tissue (tram) reconstruction was best for me. I did have a little extra tummy tissue that I could spare to share somewhere else! Thank you very much Hostess cupcakes and Twinkies. *Joy* moment!

So, in my heart I knew what I needed to do and so did my husband. It was an eight-hour surgery with a two-month recovery. So somehow I needed to schedule this surgery so it would not interfere with my daughter's senior year. I was just determined that her senior year be remembered for just that and not her mother's health or lack thereof.

Immediately, I had a peace about the surgery. I scheduled it for mid-October which was about six weeks away. I thought that would also give me time to do some early Christmas shopping and get organized so I would not stress during the long recovery. I am very detail oriented, and being an organized person, I went crazy getting everything done on my to-do list.

Every day was so full of things to do that the time was passing by so quickly. I was able to enjoy each day in the moment and not fret about the upcoming surgery. I even laughed at some of the crazy comments we heard go around.

"Did you hear, Mary is having a breast job and a tummy tuck!" Oh my, did someone actually say that! Would I actually go to this extent to have larger breasts and a flatter tummy? You have to be kidding me. But, I managed to find some laughter in it. It was actually downright hilarious because it was so absurd.

But the weeks went by quickly and finally the week of the surgery arrived. I was ready. I was totally ready!

Julia Roberts, Okay?

The night before the surgery, I remember lying in bed thinking, tomorrow they are going to cut a part of me off. Will that be brutally painful when I awake? Thank goodness there will be two new ones (breasts) in place so I don't feel disfigured. I felt like my breasts had betrayed me, and they were the enemy. I knew they had to go. Actually, I couldn't wait to get them off of me because they were detrimental to my life at this point. So, I had emotionally detached myself from them before the actual surgery even got here. I also felt it was God's way of preparing me for the surgery itself. I know my God works in mysterious ways, and I have grown to love and appreciate his ways like never before. He thinks of everything!

The day of my surgery, right before they put me to sleep, my doctor walks in and says, "Any special requests?" I wanted him to know I could be funny in the moment and responded, "Hey, can you make me look like Julia Roberts when I wake up!" It got quite a laugh.

The morning of the surgery, my husband and daughter went with me early in the morning to check into the hospital. My middle son would be up there closer to when they started the surgery, and unfortunately, my oldest son could not come home as he could not get leave. That was okay though. What he was doing was very important, and we were in no way upset. As we approached the hospital I noticed my husband and daughter were way too quiet, so of course, I had to crack a few jokes about how I was getting remodeled today! I had to make a *joy* moment for them. Though they thought I was a little crazy, I did manage to make them laugh a few times. I have to admit that part of me could not believe I was not nervous. What is the matter with me? I knew what they are getting ready to do. I knew I was having two breasts removed, a large incision, tunneling, and then a new belly button, to top it all off. I also knew I would wake up with drainage tubes everywhere and probably be very swollen. Why did I have such peace? But I did.

As we checked in, I was given my lovely hospital gown, and then they gave me a heated blanket to keep me warm as I waited to go back to surgery. Hospitals are cold and surgery rooms are even colder, so I loved my heated blanket. I learned to appreciate every little comfort when I was in the hospital!

Finally, it was time to go to surgery. I kissed everyone goodbye and slipped on a pair of special socks I wanted my doctors to notice when I arrived in surgery. As my doctor came in, he noticed them immediately. The socks said, "It's all about me today!" Since I was their only patient for the entire day (my surgery was to last between eight and nine hours), I felt those socks were appropriate. It brought in a good laugh. Mission accomplished. I gave them a *joy* moment.

The surgery required the work of two doctors. The first doctor, my actual breast surgeon, would do the double mastectomy. Then the second doctor did the reconstruction. From my understanding, both doctors were there at the beginning, but eventually the breast surgeon left once his part was complete.

Doctor number one was an older doctor, very wise, and someone that anyone would have wanted as their dad. He had great bedside manners. He was very compassionate and there to listen. I just loved this doctor and wouldn't change a thing about him.

Doctor number two was the surgeon who reconstructed, or recreated, as I like to refer to it. He was recommended by doctor number one, but he was very different from him. I had been told of his good reputation, but I didn't like his bedside manners at all. He was arrogant just like I had heard some doctors, especially plastic surgeons, could be. I didn't like him at all, but I needed him. Enough said.

God is in Control

At this point, I was lying on the operating table and getting ready to go to sleep. I was scared of going to sleep just a year before and now I welcome it like ice cream. I have learned a patient either loves it or hates it; I love it! I've had no problems with anesthesia and I love that feeling right before you go to sleep, so of course, I liked it.

As I was being prepped for surgery, I was looking at the ceiling tile and having a quiet talk to God. I remember telling him, "Okay God, this is a big surgery and you are a big God. You are in control now; take care of me." That is basically all I remember until I woke up in recovery.

While asleep, my family had many visitors in the waiting room, which was so nice since they were there all day. Some people brought up snacks for my husband and children. How very thoughtful they were! Others just sat for hours on end to help the day go by quickly for my husband and children.

The next thing I knew, I was waking up. Immediately, I was evaluating how I felt. *Hmm*, I thought. *This isn't bad; I don't have any pain.* Wow! I couldn't believe it. I slept for most of recovery. Awesome!

It was now time to go to my room. I was so ready to see my family. I wanted them to see I was doing so well. I knew the employee that wheeled my bed to my room. That was awkward to say the least. He was a young man who had been in the youth department of our church. I knew I looked pretty bad—my hair was all matted down and I had no make-up on, but who cares right now, right?

As I approached the room, I saw several church staff members there. "Hey guys, I'm doing great. I hardly have any pain." Of course everyone was probably thinking something I was not; her pain medicine had taken over! I wasn't thinking about that, so I also wasn't thinking about the fact that eventually that would wear off and then…

Oh my goodness, lots of pain! After I had been in my room for about two hours, it all hit and hit quickly. I felt like I had been run over—and several times at that. The nurses brought me morphine, but even after several shots, nothing helped. People were coming to visit, but when they saw how I was hurting, they made their visits very short. Except for one friend, she just stood there at the door and watched me cry for twenty minutes. Finally, she said her goodbyes and left.

After about three more hours of really horrible pain, the nurses realized the morphine just wasn't working for me. So, they changed my medicine to Percocet and that seemed to help. I was very good about reminding them thirty minutes before my next shot was due. I never missed a pain shot.

Once everyone left and my husband and I were alone, I found the nerve to look at my reconstruction. I was lying down and thought I would just take a peek.

I noticed two things. First of all, my breast tissue was pure white; not flesh colored like I expected. My skin looked like a porcelain doll. I later learned that it takes time for the tissue that is tunneled to look natural.

Second, as I laid there, I noticed that my reconstruction looked the same lying down or standing up. It was hilarious! I could not stop laughing. Oh Lord, you have such a sense of humor to give me a *joy* moment just then. They're not at all like I expected!

The first evening was a tough one, but it did pass and I was able to get some sleep. I knew the next day would be tough as I would need to get up and out of bed.

Early the next morning, my doctor came in about seven thirty and said, "Let's get you out of that bed." I had no idea how hard that would be. I should tell you that I had a twenty-eight-inch incision that wrapped its way from behind my waist, under my newly constructed belly button, and back around the other side of my waist. With much effort and a lot of help, the next thing I knew, I was up and sitting in the chair beside the bed. It felt nice to be sitting up, but I felt paralyzed and wondered how I would ever get back into that bed. I looked about myself and noticed five drainage tubes. I felt like a science experiment of some sort. I couldn't stand up straight long enough to look in the mirror which was probably a good thing at the time.

Family and friends came to see me. I smiled a lot and said I was doing fine, but let me tell you, I was miserable. My husband was a great help, and I needed his help constantly. He knew me well enough to know I would put up a front when visitors came so they were not aware of how truly difficult this really was. He also knew that I knew how to grit my teeth and just get through something painfully difficult by this point, so he let me just be me and continued to support and help me throughout the entire hospital stay.

I was in the hospital for four days and then released to come home. I was able to walk, but very cautiously. Just going to the bathroom was such a project. And yes, my husband literally had to help me on and off the toilet for a while even after the hospital visit. But, I knew that each day would be a little bit better and I would eventually feel normal.

Once home, I had everything set up on the couch, which is where I would dwell for the next four to six weeks. The trip home from the hospital exhausted me. Literally, I took a four hour nap when I got home. I still depended heavily on my pain pills. I didn't know enough about the good and the bad of taking these pills to care; I just didn't like the pain without them.

People came to visit a lot. I tried to hide my drainage tubes, but that was so hard to do since I had so many. I finally referred to them as "my litter." Like a cat has her litter of kitten's right there with her, that is how I felt about my drainage tubes. They were with me wherever I went. I figured I might as well joke about them and find the *joy* in it. My daughter and husband doted on me constantly. I still couldn't go to the bathroom by myself. I was amazed at how my daughter could not wait to take care of her momma, even if it meant helping me to the bathroom or draining my tubes. This was a great bonding time for us too. My drainage tubes had to be cleaned and measured several times a day. In the hospital, the nurse took care of it, so I knew I would need to do that when I got home. I got so sick to my stomach when I tried, that my husband and daughter did it for me. I just couldn't look at the fluid in the tubes.

After being home for two days, I decided to try and look at everything. No one was in the bathroom with me when I decided to look at my new body. I was totally overwhelmed when I did. I was unbelievably swollen, horribly scared, and as far as I was concerned, I looked like a freak. It didn't even look like my body anymore. It was awful. I started crying so uncontrollably that I couldn't stop. At that moment, my daughter came to the bathroom door to check on me. She saw how upset I was and called her dad to let him know he needed to come home from work. He was home in ten minutes.

I had such horrible anxiety. What had I done to myself? I chose this surgery. My body was ruined. I didn't think that I could live with this new body. It hurt, it was ugly, and it didn't feel normal at all. Nothing anyone said seemed to help. I just kept crying; I could not stop. I was so upset, I finally called both doctor's offices and talked to both nurses. They just tried to console me and tell me that I was swollen and I would look much better in a couple of weeks. I felt so out of control—so ugly.

I ended up calling a friend who was a nurse. She shared with me that what I went through was all part of the process. My body would never be the same; it would be different. She also told me that I probably felt like I had lost a part of my identity, which was a very normal process right after a surgery of this magnitude; something the doctors don't always warn you can happen. Talking with her helped some. At least I didn't feel like I was losing my mind too, and I was normal, or at least somewhat normal.

It took me a couple of days to adjust to what my reality was now. It was hard. It was very hard. It made me appreciate how God created me. His ways are perfect! That had such meaning to me now. No man could ever create like God; not even close.

All that being said, it was also hard to not clean around my home. Although my husband and children were constantly cleaning up something, I was tempted many times to do a little something around the house (when no one was looking, of course). One time, my daughter came home to check on me. When she left, I noticed how dirty the kitchen floors were. I couldn't stand it. I wet a towel, bent down, and with one hand started cleaning them. My other hand was holding my many drainage tubes. Right as I turned the corner of the kitchen, in walks my daughter again. She had forgotten something. She was simply appalled at me, and boy did I hear about it. Of course, she couldn't wait to tell her dad. Yes, I was grounded from cleaning floors for a long time after that. It became a constant joke in our house how "Mom has major surgery one day and is scrubbing floors the next!"

Weeks went by and I went to my follow-up appointments. Slowly my doctor took out the drainage tubes, one at a time. By week six, I was drainage tube free. My sister-in-law took me out to eat to celebrate. Immediate and extended family would take me to all my appointments as I could not drive yet. I was very dependent on others for quite some time—not something I enjoyed. I wasn't even tempted to disobey that rule (not driving); not with that big incision. When I was finally released to drive, I took a pillow with me everywhere I went and put it between me and the steering wheel. I just wanted to be so careful about absolutely everything!

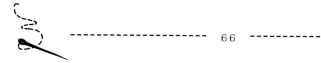

It Collapsed!

It had now been about six weeks since the surgery. I was starting to get out and do a little more, but staying within what I was told were my limitations. I still tired quite easily and would run home to rest after an hour or two away from the house.

One evening, my husband and I went to watch our daughter cheer. As I was sitting in the bleachers, I felt something weird. I wasn't sure what it was, but my stomach felt like it collapsed or something. I immediately got up and went to the bathroom to look at it myself.

As I got to the bathroom, I rushed into one of the stalls. I could not believe what I saw. My belly button had a huge hole right next to it. I could see my insides. It made me sick to look at. I actually had a hole, about one and a half inches in diameter, right next to my belly button. I guess the tissue just caved in to the point of tearing loose and left a gash of tissue showing. It was utterly scary to me. I was standing there looking at it and all I could think was, *I am like one of those people they show on TV who had had a surgery gone bad.*

I immediately covered myself up and went back to the bleachers to tell my husband. As much as I tried to explain what it looked like, he couldn't really get the picture until we got home and I showed him. He was speechless and very upset!

It was hard to sleep that night. I knew I would call my doctor first thing in the morning, but it was hard to lie there in bed and not be sick over what was happening to my body. I felt like a freak, again. I felt gross. Little did I know that this was the beginning of a *lot* of problems from my surgery.

The next morning finally came. I called the doctor the minute they opened for the day. My doctor was out doing surgery all day. After explaining what had happened the night before, the nurse insisted I come in and see his partner. I was okay with that.

My husband had an easy work schedule that day so he was able to come with me. It made it easier for me, knowing that he would be with me that day. I was almost embarrassed to show this doctor my stomach because I felt so ugly. As I showed the doctor, he didn't say much other than I had an infection (probably internal) that caused this to happen. I did watch as he looked at the nurse really weird once he saw my infection. I have often wondered what was said after I left that day. The only solution for now was to put a compound solution and gauze on it. He explained what this solution was and where to get the prescription filled as I could not just go to any pharmacy for a compound solution. So off we went to get it filled. After filling the prescription, I read that it was 90 percent Clorox and 10 percent alcohol. That was a little scary to me. I must have had some infection! So basically, I was to put Clorox in my infection to dry it out. That's just so very wrong as far as I am concerned, but I did it just like I was told.

There are no words to describe how awful it was to doctor this infection. The doctor had me cutting long strips of gauze and soaking it in the compound and then filling that hole in my stomach with it. I had to do that every couple of hours. It smelled so bad, and it smelt ten times worse when I would take it out. I was now officially the grossest person I had ever met. I was in tears every time I looked at it or cleaned it out. The doctor said that this solution would dry it out and it would close itself. I assumed that would happen and it would look okay afterwards. How could I have possibly thought that?

Weeks and weeks went by and it just never seemed to get better. I had a scheduled appointment with my actual doctor for two weeks from when it collapsed, and he too said it would just take time.

I think it is fair to say that I just trusted my doctor until something went wrong and even then, I just assumed this happens sometimes.

Finally, a month went by, and I realized I was not getting better. My belly button didn't look one bit better. As a matter a fact, I didn't feel right. I felt sick to my stomach sometimes and was having fevers off and on.

In the middle of all this, I was somewhat sidetracked because my son was coming in from the Army on leave for Christmas and I wanted to be able to enjoy our two weeks with him. We didn't get to see him much since he joined the military, and this time was very important to not just my husband and me but also, his brother, sister, and his son. I didn't want anything medical to spoil our time.

I chose to kind of ignore how I felt the week before Christmas and focus on family time. That was fine at first, but the day after Christmas I could no longer take the discomfort I was feeling. I remember realizing I could no longer ignore how sick I felt. I was lying on the couch every night the week before, suffering through the discomfort and fever and curling up in a ball thinking I might die of some stupid infection because of the way I felt. I had also started to notice a big lump or swelling right under my left breast and my incision had a small area opening up on it too. I decided it was time to call my doctor. Their offices were closed because the twenty-sixth fell over the weekend, but he was on call so he answered. He seemed quite concerned and asked if I could get to the office and he would meet me there. Of course, with the help of my husband, I was there in twenty minutes.

I am appalled and disgusted at what happened next. My husband was in the waiting room as I went back to one of the patient rooms. I was lying on the patient table and the next thing I knew, as the doctor was checking my stomach, all I could see was blood. I have had a less than normal feeling so what I didn't realize was he had a tool that he had inserted in my belly button that he was using to probe for fluid up towards my breast. He thought maybe the swelling under my breast was fluid and he could get to it. I was sick to my stomach at his approach. To this day, I do not believe that was any way to handle my problems. He finally looked at me and said, "I think I will need to schedule you for surgery (exploratory), that way I can check what the swelling is, re-do your belly button, and fix your incision."

How could I not see that I had a bad infection that was causing all these problems? How could my doctor not see that before it got to this point either? He told me he had to call the hospital and see when the operating room was available, but he wanted me to have surgery as soon as possible. The soonest time was on the twenty-ninth at nine in the morning. Of course, I scheduled it, but it was upsetting to me because my son had to catch a plane at eleven in the morning that day so I would have to say goodbye to him as I was going into surgery. Not ideal at all.

The next few days went by slowly and all this put such a damper on the holidays with our family, but I did feel ready for the surgery on the twenty-ninth as we drove up. I physically felt so bad that I knew I had to do something. It made no sense to me that I wasn't afraid of dying of cancer, but I did have great concern of dying from an infection.

I said my goodbyes to my family and son who had to get to the airport and was rolled away to the operating room.

I didn't have my great sense of humor about me that day; I wasn't cracking jokes as I lay there waiting to be put to sleep. I remember looking at the ceiling thinking, *Here I am, Lord. Though I still have no fear thanks to you, I do wonder this time, will I wake up from this or meet*

you sooner than expected? I am totally in your hands and I know that full well.

As I was laying there waiting to be put to sleep, my doctor walked in and was talking to me. Though I may have heard this wrong, I am almost for sure I heard him say, "I just need to get in there and see what is going on and figure out what that lump is under your breast." Hearing that put the thought of more cancer in my head right as they put me to sleep. Not a peaceful way to go to sleep. Thank goodness for my relationship with Christ!

Waking Up

Two and a half hours went by. I woke up to the nurse pulling the tube out of my throat. Wow! That was no way to wake up. She was very apologetic and said typically they can get that out before the patient is alert enough to know what just happened. Oops! But that was okay; my pain seemed very manageable so I was not going to complain.

I had to stay in recovery for about an hour and a half, but it was much better than the last surgery. I remembered sleeping a lot—just waking up as the nurse checked my vitals.

The next thing I knew, it was time to go to my hospital room.

Anyhow, I was anxious to get to my room and see what I look like. As soon as the nurse left the room, I sat up as best I could to take a look. My incision looked normal, the swelling under my breast looked much better, and I had a new belly button—that would be belly button number three for me. I wasn't sure if I liked the way it looked though. The skin all around it looked wrinkled and funny to me, but at least there wasn't a hole beside it.

Later that day my doctor came in and said all went well. He said the swelling was caused by scar tissue that he removed and also that he cleaned out everything and put some kind of a liquid antibiotic all over to kill the infection. He seemed happy with the results. I did not say anything about my belly button at the time. For some reason I was uncomfortable to address it in the midst of everything else that had gone wrong.

I went home the next day as they wanted to keep me one night to make sure I was really doing okay. A one night hospital stay was a breeze for me, and it went by fast. I even slept well that night since I didn't have all the discomforts as before the surgery. I did have two drainage tubes that went home with me. Yuck!

Again, I was given instructions on my limited activity. The couch is slowly but surely becoming my best friend. I have well learned that the body does heal, it just takes time.

During all this time, my dad was also battling cancer, and it was starting to get worse. I still felt I could never complain because I was able to cut my cancer off and my dad could not. It helped me keep perspective whenever I would even consider having a pity moment for myself.

Life Becomes Normal

Six weeks after surgery, I felt good—good enough to do something, so I started to look for a job. I felt that my life was going back to normal. I found an awesome job working for a staffing agency and felt that life was finally moving on from my cancer and the problems related to the surgery. I felt like it was a chapter finally closed in my life, and I was very ready for that.

After working for about three or four months, I noticed something peculiar. I had a lump, or more of a bulge, right in the middle below my chest. It was hard and felt very uncomfortable. I even noticed sometimes that I had shortness of breath and thought maybe it was related to that bulge.

Two months went by before I made a doctor appointment, but in all honestly, the bulge was not noticeable consistently so it took me a little time to realize I needed to address it. During this time, my dad took a sudden turn for the worse and died. We knew he wasn't well and knew he would probably die that year, but we really weren't expecting him to die when he did. This threw me for a loop to say the least, so by the time I finally went in to see a doctor, it was late June—about a month after Dad died.

As I went back to the patient room, I do remember the nurse asking me a lot of questions about the bulge. It was very noticeable to her too. I was at a place in my life where everything was hard because I really missed my dad a lot. When the doctor came in, he didn't have much compassion. He was a bit harsh when he felt the bulge and told me it was just scar tissue and I needed to massage that area more. Part of my initial recovery was to massage the stomach area to help promote the healing process. He gave me about two minutes and left. I remember thinking, *What a waste of time that was.* When he left the nurse started making excuses for his behavior and I just cried and said, "I doubt that I will ever come back to him, *ever!*" I ended up telling her I was going through an emotional time as my dad had just died of cancer, and I couldn't handle that doctor today. She understood, I could just tell. She didn't have to say too much.

I drove home that day making a commitment to myself that I would never grace that office or that doctor ever again. I kept that commitment. I never did.

Suck it Up!

I am not a fan of the expression "suck it up," but it per-fectly fits what I did. I massaged that bulge for three months thinking I had pampered myself too much, and it would eventually subside. After all this time, I thought I had learned to tolerate pain and discomfort more, but I was beginning to doubt that. How sad.

It was now October, and the bulge was definitely worse than better. I was so uncomfortable with it. At night I would lay on the couch to watch TV with my husband and you could see the bulge through my shirt. It was uncomfortable all the time. Finally, I decided I would go to my primary doctor and get his opinion. It was time for an annual check-up and I respected his opinion. I made an appointment for the next week and, yes, waited.

The day of the appointment arrived, and my doc-tor immediately said, "That is not right; something is wrong." His first thought was that it was an ulcer. So he put me on medicine to help get control of it. After a month of that, he realized it must be something else because the bulge continued to grow. I actually was starting to look disfigured. Though it wasn't funny, sometimes I would look in the mirror and just laugh at how I looked. I can laugh until I cry. God gave me, as well as both of my parents, that trait because he knew I would need it someday.

So, I went back to my doctor. He was concerned that maybe it was my gall bladder. So he set up some tests and said to make an appointment with him after they were done. This took a couple of weeks, and when I returned to my doctor, I learned my gall bladder was fine. He was a bit puzzled because he felt sure that was what it was. In the meantime, the bulge seemed to be getting worse and worse. *What is the matter with me?* I thought. I didn't know anyone who had problems like me. I just wanted someone to help me get rid of it—whatever it was.

Next, the doctor set me up for an MRI. This took another couple of weeks to get in for the test and get the results. It was now mid-January and all I could think was, *Last Christmas, I felt miserable with all the problems from my surgery. Now a year has gone by, and I have a whole new set of problems. Why can't I just get healthy? What is the matter with me?*

Once the MRI was complete, I went back to my primary doctor so we could go over the results. To my surprise, I had an abdominal hernia. Not just one, but two of them. He said I would need surgery. *Oh, what the heck. Why not? Another year, another surgery. I am becoming the surgery queen.* We joked about this at home.

We set up the surgery for a few weeks later. It would be the first part of March. This gave me enough time to get some things in order at home and at work. I had been dealing with those hernias for quite some time, so waiting a few more weeks wasn't going to hurt anything.

By this point, I had it down. I knew how to set up my post-surgery, stuck-on-the-couch supplies—tissues, magazines, meds, etc.—and prepare myself for recovery.

One luxury I always allowed myself was a new pair of pajamas each time I went into the hospital for surgery. I was beginning to have quite a nice collection of them. I didn't care for the hospital gowns, as most people don't, so I managed to get out of the hospital gown and into my own pajamas pretty quickly once I got into my room.

This surgery was a laparoscopic surgery, so I thought this one would be a walk in the park compared to my other surgeries. Five little cuts compared to a long incision. That just had to be easier.

The one thing this lapse in time did do for me was made me think a bit too. If I would have been diagnosed properly last June, maybe it would have only been the one hernia. It got worse as time went by. How sad that my doctor made light of my concerns and didn't catch that, especially because it is a known fact that the tunneling process done during my surgery is known to sometimes cause the stomach wall to weaken and cause hernias. How in the world did he not diagnose me correctly when I went in to have it checked?

I wasn't anxious about this surgery. I was just very ready to have it done and be out of this discomfort. The surgery was set up for two in the afternoon on a Tuesday. I decided to go ahead and work until eleven that morning and have my husband pick me up and take me directly to the hospital. I thought if I kept myself busy it would help me to not think about the fact that I could not eat or drink anything after midnight. The not eating doesn't bother me; I can handle that. But the not drinking anything at all literally drives me crazy. It's like I got so incredibly thirsty all because I couldn't have a drink. So, I knew I needed to be busy to help me get to middle of the day.

The morning went a little slow, but finally eleven o'clock arrived and my husband picked me up from work. We actually joked all the way to the hospital—another day, another surgery, another *joy* moment for us.

As we arrived, I had to laugh. I knew this routine completely. I knew not to bring any jewelry, to bring my own socks (I like them better than the hospital socks), and to ask for heated blankets. Hospitals are so cold, and since I tend to get a little nervous before surgery, warm blankets seemed to help sooth me. I was quite used to all the typical questions and then a visit from the doctor and anesthesiologist. Then I sat and waited…and waited. Fortunately, the wait was only thirty minutes, and off I went after a kiss and a prayer from my husband. We opted not to tell many people about this surgery. First of all, we felt I would be home the next day and that I would heal quickly since this sounded like a pretty basic surgery compared to some of my previous surgeries. Second, we just didn't feel like telling everyone that I was having another surgery.

The surgery took about an hour and a half. When I woke up in recovery, I was caught quite off guard by how uncomfortable I was. I was in so much pain. *Wait*

a minute, I thought. *This is supposed to be an easy surgery. What's the deal?* After another hour and a half in recovery, they finally let me go to my room. My doctor came in to tell me, not only were there two hernias, but they found a third one. He then went on to tell me that he had to do quite a bit of work to fix all three of them. No wonder I felt so bad. I also learned that it didn't really matter how much a doctor had to cut on you on the outside. What really mattered was how much they had to do to fix you on the inside. It was a tough lesson to learn, but it made so much sense in that moment.

Due to the amount of surgery he did, my doctor decided to keep me in the hospital for a couple of days and on liquids to give my insides time to heal.

I had the pleasure of Jell-O and broth, but I also had the added pleasure of what looked like mud pie with my dinner meal. When I asked what it was each night, they said it was ground up meat of some sort. No matter how hungry I was, I could not bring myself to eat that. I just looked at it. It smelled too gross to put in my mouth. My nurse was not very pleased with me. She gave me the same look of disapproval when she came to pick up my tray each evening. It was hard to get out of bed because my chest and abdomen hurt like crazy. Finally on Friday, day four of the hospital visit, I talked them into letting me have a normal breakfast. I was starving at that point. I needed food—real food. I enjoyed that meal so much; it tasted so good! I think those were the best eggs and bacon I have ever eaten. But after four days of that liquid diet, I so appreciated hospital food!

I was released from the hospital late that Friday afternoon. I was so ready to go home. This was a much longer visit than I anticipated, and I had only brought one pair of pajamas.

Once home, I noticed something funny. I looked down at my hand and sure enough, the nurse forgot to take out my IV. My husband and I just started laughing because we both knew I would not go back to have it taken out. Yes, I took it out myself. At this point, I had watched nurses take them out enough that it was a no brainer. I had it out and covered with a band-aid in a matter of seconds. Such *joy*. My husband and I thought it was too funny!

I was so glad to be home. I took a pain pill and gladly went right to my recovery couch and took a wonderful, uninterrupted, three-hour-long nap. That was the best sleep I had had in days, and I was thankful to be home and done with surgery, again.

As the evening arrived, I started to feel pretty miserable. The one meal had made me miserable. Without embarrassing myself too much, I needed to go to the bathroom, but just couldn't. This is one of the reasons the doctors like to keep you in the hospital a few days. Let's face it; they want to know that your bowels are working. Mine weren't. I had a lot of pain that was all right in my abdomen. I was in tears. *How can gas pain be so uncomfortable*, I thought. But it was. I even called a friend of mine that was a nurse to get advice. She gave me advice on things I could take that would eventually ease my pain and discomfort. I had my husband go to the store and grab everything she suggested.

It took about a day and a half to get out of that pain. It was not fun and not something I would want to do ever again. Gas pain and abdominal surgery do not make for a good mix. Trust me. I don't know if you have been counting or not, but I have done this several times by now.

I stayed home for about five more days and decided to try and go back to work. I lasted hours that first day, and then I went to half days for another week. I still needed a pain pill about half way through the day, so I would work until noon and then take a pill on my way home. By the time I arrived home, the pill would be starting to take affect and I would head for my favorite couch and take a nap. This went on for about ten days and then I was able to work as normal.

It was during this time that I realized how tired I always felt. I just didn't feel like I had ever totally recovered from all this surgery. I was just so tired all the time. After talking to my husband and praying together, we decided it was time for a drastic change in my life. I was going to quit my job and just focus on me. I had talked about writing a book about my experience with both of my parents during their battle with cancer and their deaths. I was going to start that. I felt really good about this decision. I gave a two week notice and was done. It was a very long two weeks because I could hardly wait for this new chapter of my life. I was done with all that surgery and anxious to retire and write.

Retired and Loving it!

At first I wasn't doing much writing. I just loved getting up, lounging around the house, doing my devotional and sipping on coffee. Everyone would be out early and it was just so quiet and peaceful. I physically was feeling better very quickly because so much stress was out of my life.

After about a month I realized, I had not written a word. Had I taken on a task that was above me? I had no idea. I had to make myself sit down finally and start writing. I was concerned as to how hard it would be to recall everything I went through with my parents, but it was amazing how every little bit of it came back to me.

I got to where I loved my writing days. I would kiss everyone goodbye as they left for their day, grab my cup of coffee, and go to the computer room. I would be there for five and six hours some days, sometimes crying over the keyboard as I relived those memories. But it was very comforting. It actually helped me as I was still dealing with the pain from my dad's death months earlier.

So that was my life for the next six months. I would stay home and write one day and get out and play the next. It was very healing for me both spiritually and physically. It was a decision very well made, and I knew it. I was also very proud of myself for actually, *finally*, writing like I said I would.

A Price for Comfort

Six months had passed since my hernia surgery. Though I had healed from this surgery, I still had so many discomforts that I just didn't really want to deal with. I just figured I was stuck with these discomforts. When my initial reconstruction was done, there were some not so perfect results.

After my surgery, things did not look like I expected. First of all, one breast was two sizes larger than the other. That is very noticeable and challenging when buying a bra. Do you buy too big and stuff one side or do you buy too small and be squished?

I also had a very ugly belly button. The first one, the one God gave me, was perfect. The second one, the one my doctor gave me, was high and to the left. It was awkward. Then, when that one collapsed, the third one was okay except it had a big, wrinkled scar about two inches all the way around it. It was not a pretty sight at all.

I also had scar tissue that was very hard and uncomfortable underneath my left breast. It would get more sore as the day went on.

Lastly, my waist was not the same. The way I had been sewed up left it very uncomfortable for me to wear pants with buttons. Regular pants hurt me around my waist and by my belly button. It made me mad that I had to wear elastic pants. That was unacceptable to me.

So, in the back of my mind, I knew I had a decision to make—to address the discomforts and consider more surgery, or to live uncomfortably. I did not want to think about this, but the last six months allowed me to heal as much as possible, and I knew it was time to make this decision.

By this point, I was not afraid of surgery. I knew the only way past the discomforts was the one thing I had grown accustomed to—surgery. I also knew it couldn't hurt to at least go talk to a doctor and see what he would say about it all. So, of course, I decided to move forward and search for a new surgeon—a new plastic surgeon, that is.

As I started calling doctors in town, I was surprised how many wouldn't do a corrective surgery from a tram operation. Actually, there were only five doctors that would consider it that were within my insurance plan. Of two of the five doctors on my list, I had heard some not-so-good, horror stories so I immediately marked them off the list. The third doctor was not interested after seeing the results of my tram surgery. He was honest and said he wasn't comfortable performing a corrective surgery on me. There were just two doctors left on my list to consider. I was beginning to think that God was shutting the door, and I was just supposed to live with the discomforts I was having from the initial surgery. As I made an appointment to meet with the fourth doctor on my list, I did not get my hopes up for him to want to try and correct my concerns. I figured he would say the same thing as the third doctor that I had been in to see just weeks earlier.

The day of the appointment arrived, and I prepared myself for another awkward time to have to show all my imperfections to yet another person, and a man at that. It didn't matter if I knew the doctor had seen many undressed bodies before, this was my body and it was very personal to me. It also didn't help that my body didn't even look close to its' original form.

So, here I go. As I arrived at the office, I must say, I loved his staff—from the receptionist, to the nurse, to his assistant. They were just so genuinely nice and sincere in how they asked questions and handled all the basic information they needed. Then the doctor came in the room. He was an older man, which, for some reason, I really liked because I feel they have more experience and wisdom at that point in their life. Plus, I figure they have seen it all by now. We talked about me for quite some time before he asked me to show him my discomforts and concerns. He made it quite clear that he had seen results like mine many times before and he could fix all of them. It took all I had not to throw my arms around him and cry all over him. But I didn't, I just very politely said, "Awesome, let's do it."

Because I need to plan everything (my husband and children know this all too well), I decided to wait until after Christmas as I wanted to not worry about being less than 100 percent for the holidays. Christmas is my favorite holiday, and I had way too much on my mind. I had to finish gift shopping, decorating, and, my favorite part of it all, baking all my Christmas goodies!

So, without even asking any specifics on the surgery, I said, "Let's do this after the first of the year." As I left the doctor's office, I made an appointment to come back in January to finalize all the specifics for the surgery.

I went home that day so delighted. I knew that how I felt was temporary and it would change. I was so happy for that. I thought, *Thank you, God, for leading me to this doctor.* I didn't even need to meet with the fifth doctor on the list. I knew this was the right doctor without a doubt.

Needless to say, I threw myself into the holidays as usual and was able to enjoy every moment, discomfort and all.

But Doctor...

The holidays were over, the tree and decorations were down, and everyone had gone back to their schedules. I was happy I had decided to allow myself the holidays plus a week or two to clean up from them. What a perfect time to plan my doctor appointment to prepare for my upcoming surgery.

I was actually excited to see the staff again. I just felt like they knew me, even though they didn't. Little did I know, they would get to know me over the next year.

When the doctor came in to go over the surgery, I had no idea what he was getting ready to say. I must be clueless or something, but I hadn't even thought about what, specifically, he might need to do to actually fix everything.

As I was sitting on the table, he began to tell me the process of the surgery he was getting ready to perform. He said, "I will first need to turn you over on your stomach, do liposuction, to correct the tissue on both sides of your waste. Then after we turn you back over, I will need to open up the old incision and redo the one breast to make it smaller. I will then redo your belly button and then repair or replace your mesh covering your hernias. Finally, I will then sew you up differently so your waist will be more comfortable in your clothing." The new incision would be longer as he would have to cut a little more.

I was speechless at first. I finally managed to ask, "How long will this surgery take to finish?"

He said, "About nine hours." As I sat there totally shocked by all I had just heard, I wanted to cry. I honestly didn't think I could go through all that again. Then he went on to say I would be down for six to eight weeks with five drainage tubes. That was what almost put me over the edge. I finally had to admit to him that I had no idea that it would be that much surgery. I guess I was so excited that he said he could fix everything, I just didn't think about what the process of doing that might include. I was so upset but did a pretty good job of hiding it until he gave me pre-surgery instructions and sent me on my way. I had ten days before the surgery to prepare myself.

Even though I was quite upset at everything he would need to do, I did find one thing funny (I guess I could call it another joy moment). I was going to have yet another belly button.

As I drove away, as upset as I was about it all, I knew I was going to put myself through this. I wanted to feel normal and comfortable again and I knew I was willing to take on all that pain and discomfort to get it back. *I am a fighter, and I am not going to stop until I feel I have completely won this battle. If feeling normal is part of the fight, then I must take on this challenge again.*

Surgery Again

The next ten days went by pretty quickly. I am one of those people that once my mind was set on something, I was ready to do it and be done. I bought two new pajama outfits as I knew I would be in the hospital several days.

We actually made light of this surgery to our children because we wanted them to stay at school. Plus, it was an optional surgery that I chose to do. My biggest concern was that it was a long surgery that would require a long recovery to go with it.

So, early that morning in mid-January, my husband and I went to the hospital for the typical routine we call surgery. The nurses asked their routine questions, gave me the routine gown, and gave me the routine, no-jewelry-during-surgery talk. They asked Joe to move his car once I went to surgery again—all routine. I was pretty calm as I knew this would eventually make me more comfortable.

When the doctor came in to draw on me for my surgery, I did ask if I could have a pain pump put in this time. He was great and said, "Absolutely, there is no reason for you to have any pain you don't need." No wonder I liked this doctor so much. I knew over the past couple years I had learned to tolerate pain more, but that didn't mean I liked it any better. I knew that the less pain I felt, the more rest I would get, and the quicker I would heal. My doctor also told me that at the end of the surgery they would give me a medicine boost for pain so I would not wake up miserable in recovery. I really liked this doctor. The thought of waking up without pain was almost too good to believe. I thought to myself, *let's just see if it works!*

The time came to go to surgery, and I was ready. I knew this routine way too well. They asked me to move onto the surgery table, that very narrow table made for skinny people. I knew to lay my arms out (like on a cross). They strapped them down and started to set up my arm with the IV in it for my anesthesia. I actually enjoyed the next couple of minutes. Is it sad that I was so ready for that relaxed feeling because then I really wouldn't care? I felt so good for a few seconds. And then I was out.

The moment of truth was here. They had just woken me up from this long surgery, and I had a moment to recollect my thoughts. *How do I feel?* I thought for only a moment. *Oh my goodness, I have little to no pain. Thank you, Lord. I am sure there will be pain in the next few days and weeks, but thank you for sparing me that when I first woke up. I can do this.*

I felt so good I just kept going back to sleep. I'm sure the anesthesia wasn't helping me stay awake either. I wanted to go to a regular room, but the nurse said I needed to be able to stay awake a little more. It took me an hour or so to come out of it enough, but I finally did and was taken to my room. My husband was waiting for me there and it was nice to know the surgery was done. Now all I had to do was heal one day at a time.

Post Surgery

One thing I have learned over the past few years is that every visit to the hospital is different. It all depends on your surgery, your pain, and the people who are there to help you. Sometimes it goes very well and sometimes not.

On the day after surgery, my husband and I were walking the halls very slowly as part of the healing process. As we were getting back to my room a nurse passed by and said, "I just have to tell you that I like your pajamas better this year than last year!" *Am I here so often that they know my buy-a-new-pair-of-pajamas policy each time I have surgery.* I looked at my husband and said, "I know I have been here too much for her to notice that." We both actually thought it was hilarious (joy moment) the more we thought about it.

Post surgery was very hard this time. Even after all I had been told about the surgery prior to having it, I was unprepared for how beat up my body would feel and look. The first day, after my boost of medicine wore off, I could not get comfortable. My backside hurt as much as my front. I could not understand why I hurt so bad on the backside, so I had my husband look at it. His eyes said it all. I was black and blue from my shoulders to my lower back from the liposuction. Come to find out, it took the doctor two hours of liposuction to correct my waist. Even though I was glad he did what he needed to do, I was very uncomfortable. I pressed my pain pump frequently—very frequently. I was not stupid, and I knew that it would only release so much medicine no matter how often I pressed it, but I still pressed it often just in case it accidently gave me more than it should. It was hard to get comfortable when I had surgery on both my front and backside.

I learned that even though hospitals pride themselves on keeping me out of pain that does not necessarily happen. I noticed that my pain pump quit working. When I asked the nurse about it, she was polite but said there was nothing she could do. As the day went on, I really was hurting quite a bit. By seven in the evening, I could hardly stand the pain. I was tense and trembling by that point. Another shift of nurses had come on and I asked the new nurse what she thought, she checked the pump closely and noticed it was no longer connected to my IV. So I had gone all day without medicine. That could have been prevented if the first nurse would have been more thorough. This nurse was great; she could not put the pump back in so she gave me a shot that would take away my pain more quickly than a pain pill. She made sure to bring in my pain medicine every four hours throughout the night. She knew my rest was an important part of my healing process. The next two days were brutal. Getting out of bed was not fun—it hurt. It hurt a lot. But the more I made myself get up, the better I felt. And I knew that meant I would hopefully go to the bathroom so I could go home.

Yes, I had to go number one and number two before I could go home. Of course, this was not something patients like to talk about, but it was a very important part of the healing process. It is also important to know that after abdominal surgery, going number two was never fun. It was a very painful process.

My body did not like going to the bathroom and took longer than most to do its duties. So, on the second day, the nurse recommended I take no pain meds as they constipate me and maybe then I could go. Nothing happened all day. I had pain, but I knew it was best to deal with the pain so I could go. By night time the nurse gave me something to drink to help me go. It was the worst thing I have ever had to drink in my life. It took me an entire hour to get it down. I waited and nothing happened again. All night long, I never went to sleep; I had a lot of pain, and never went to the bathroom. I was beginning to hit my peak of what I could handle when the nurse came back into my room. I told her I had to take a pain pill because I was so tense at this point, I could no longer do it. The next shift nurse suggested I drink another one of those awful drinks. As much as I didn't want to, I agreed and finished it within 30 minutes. Finally, about three hours later, I was able to go to the bathroom. Of course, I was sitting on the toilet crying like a baby with how much my body hurt for that, but mission accomplished. I did it.

The doctor wanted me to stay one more night, which was fine by me. I was going to get to go home and it had only been four days. I felt good. I had done it. Mission accomplished. I had pushed myself to have that big surgery so I could hopefully enjoy feeling normal once again. I knew it would be at least a few months until my body would get there, but the worst was over with for me.

Patience Mary!

For some reason I was less patient this time. I was so ready to heal and move on from all this in my life. I wanted to look normal, or should I say more normal, and feel better. When one has had as many stitches and scars as I have, normal is never what it used to be. I have scars from my chest to my hips; scars from things taken out, things that were moved around, new things that were created, and of course from the many drainage tubes I had throughout the surgeries. I refer to these scars as old battle wounds because I truly believe it was a battle and I fought hard to win that battle.

My doctor was a very good doctor and wanted to make sure he did not take out my drainage tubes too early. Since infections have haunted me a bit, my doctor was very slow to take even one out. There were five total. I would go to post-op visits every week. Finally, after the fourth week post surgery, he agreed to take out one of them. Then each week following, he would take one more out. Finally, after eight weeks post surgery, I was drainage-tube free. The swelling was going down, and I could definitely see and feel the difference. My doctor also took out scar tissue on the side of my left breast which made me so much more comfortable. I had an adorable new belly button—it was small and had no wrinkles around it and it was actually right in the center of my stomach. I could finally wear pants that button, and they were not uncomfortable. I'd done it! I made a decision to fight for more comfort, and I did what it took to get there. I was pretty proud of myself because it was just an option—nothing I had to do. God is good because he watched over me and helped me through this.

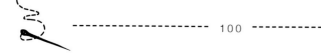

Let's face it, when I had the mastectomy, the doctor did take my nipples too during the mastectomy surgery. I actually had a "skin-sparing mastectomy which meant they took all my inside tissue and the nipple, but left my breast skin. It was important for them to take my nipples because my cancer was inside a milk duct and therefore, keeping my nipples would have given me a bigger chance of getting my cancer back.

Nipple reconstruction is completely optional. Early on I had decided it was not something I would need to mess with because who would know anyhow. Plus, I didn't like the options for nipple reconstruction.

The first option is where the doctor actually re-creates a nipple using tissue from another part of my body. One thing I have learned is that when a doctor takes tissue from another part of my body, it leaves a funny sensation to that part of me. I know how it feels when my hand is asleep. Well, that is similar to how it feels when they take tissue from an area. One area they take tissue from, for example, is my bottom and I didn't want a funny sensation every time I sat down. I just wasn't interested in any additional discomforts. Remember, The goal was not just to look normal, but to feel normal as well. Plus, when they actually create a nipple, it cannot function like a real nipple. Unfortunately, it is always erect. Now that was the last thing I would need to be worrying about. I would be so self-conscious of that all the time. I have never been one to bring attention to myself and I wasn't about to start.

The next option was tattooing a nipple onto the breast. At the beginning that just didn't appeal to me either. I am not big on tattoos, so the jokes in our house were pretty funny "Hey, guess what?" my children would say. "We can't have tattoos, but Mom can!" Or they would say, "Mom, instead of a nipple, why don't you have a tattoo that says 'I (heart symbol) Joe'." Needless to say, they were having a lot of fun at my expense.

Neither one of these options interested me, so early on I decided it was one surgery or procedure I would not have to bother with.

Oddly enough, after I had the corrective surgery on everything, I had a change of heart. I guess part of me decided that I had come this far, let's complete the entire process of looking and feeling normal. I decided to discuss it with my doctor at one of my post-op appointments. I actually became determined to go through with it. I opted for the tattooing as I felt I would look more normal.

The day came for this procedure. I was not nervous at all. My doctor said I would be somewhat awake for it; I was okay with that. I did have to go into the hospital for it, but it was an out-patient procedure that took an hour with a minimal recovery time. My husband came with me because he would need to take me home since I would not be able to drive afterwards.

It was quite funny to think about it. I went into the operating room without nipples and came out with them. As the doctor started the process, I did not like being awake for it after all. I could hear and smell everything. I was too close to seeing as they were creating a tattoo and burning my skin. As he began the surgery, I told him I wasn't doing as well with being awake as I thought I would do, so he put me to sleep. I woke up feeling fine; no pain. My chest was wrapped up so I couldn't really see what I looked like. He gave me some instructions and sent me home.

Of course, I went immediately to the bathroom to see what I looked like once we arrived home. I had little bandages over each breast. I was quite shocked to see two bloody circles with darker circles in the middle of them. It looked so sore. I was so grateful that I didn't have a lot of feeling in my breast anymore. Like every other surgery or procedure I'd had before, I knew things would look different after a few weeks. Thank goodness, because at first I looked like I had been in an accident and burned myself. It did take weeks to heal. I was limited on the clothing I could wear also. It was a pain, but I knew how to deal with it. And there were no drainage tubes so I wasn't going to complain.

It actually took at least a month for them to heal and it was summer time so I was able to adjust my wardrobe accordingly. Once all was healed I was not happy with how they looked. They didn't look like breasts with nipples; they looked like breasts with circles tattooed on them. They didn't look even close to normal. I felt a little bit like a freak.

So, I made an appointment to go back to the doctor and see what we could do to make them look more normal. The nice thing for me was that I was so comfortable with this doctor at this point that I felt I could tell him anything and he would understand. He was a very good listener and had such compassion about him.

The day of the appointment arrived. By now, it was late summer. After looking at the results, he encouraged me to let him do a procedure that would make them look more natural. He created a way to cut the tissue right on the breast and create a nipple from that tissue. He would cut a cross-shaped incision in the center of the breast (for me that would be right in the middle of my tattoo), invert the tissue and form a nipple. At first, I was not interested because I was afraid it would show through my clothes. He told me he would make them very small, and I would not have to worry about it. After going back and forth, I decided to look at my options. I could look tattooed and unnatural the rest of my life or take one more chance to look normal. I knew I had to do the surgery.

We set it up for two weeks later. I was very ready to get this over with because I knew it would be at least a month of healing time. I felt like there was always another surgery in the picture, and I knew this should finally be the end of it. So having my "do it all" personality, I thought, *Let's get it done.*

The day of the surgery arrived. It was the same routine—my husband took me in, they put me to sleep so

I didn't have to watch any of it, I had a short recovery afterward, and I went home.

Of course, I wanted to see what it looked like as soon as I arrived home. This time when I took the bandages off, I started laughing out loud. There were 2 cone-shaped objects over my breast. Another joy moment. I laughed so hard, I was actually crying. I called the nurse and she told me I needed to keep them there for a week or so to help the nipples stay in place. Now what in the world do I wear to not look to obvious now? The next day I needed to be at church for a meeting and I must have tried on thirty tops before I found one that hid everything. I also made the mistake of looking under the cones to see how my nipples looked. They were huge; or at least huge compared to what I was expecting to see. Immediately, my emotions took over, and I started crying uncontrollably. *This is not how I wanted to look. What have I done to myself? Can I undo this?*

I tried to pull myself together to go to my meeting. As I walked into church a friend stopped me and asked how my surgery went. I had told just a few people about it, and she was one of them. I guess I had hit my emotional peak because I burst into tears and ran out of the church. I had all this anxiety about making such a big mistake and being stuck looking like this.

My emotions were running rampant. I called my doctor's office crying as I sat outside the church. The receptionists got the nurse as the doctor was with a patient. I cried all over myself; she could hardly understand a thing I said. I actually remember that I told her something like, "I looked like the wrong kind of girl!"

It took her a while to calm me down. She reminded me that I was swollen and it would look very different in time. I was still pretty upset, so she had me hold while she went and talked to the doctor. When she came back, she said the doctor suggested I take the cones off and put pressure on the nipples to make them lay more flat and they would look like real nipples. I was told to do that frequently for the next two days until I came back in for my post-op visit.

I walked around my house pressing on my nipples every chance I could get. Now is that just wrong or what? I had to explain to my children what I was doing so they wouldn't think I was weird. We are a family who likes to joke about things, so we all had a good time with this. Yes, we definitely refer to this as another joy moment. At this point, I am sure my family had agreed on one thing for sure, "Our Mom has lost it; she is no longer normal; she's crazy! But, at least she knows when to laugh, right?"

A few days went by, and I could tell quite a difference from putting pressure on my nipples. When I went in to see my doctor, he was happy with how things were looking. He sent me home for another month to heal. Though I was limited on clothing options again, I managed to get through that month, and slowly, I noticed that I started to look normal. I could finally say I had two breasts with normal looking nipples.

The Unexpected

Several months passed after my final nipple reconstruction. It was late fall. Time and life seemed to finally move on from my journey with cancer and all the surgeries and procedures that followed.

Right after thanksgiving I noticed my incision looked irritated. Within a weeks' time it seemed to get worse each day. At first, I thought it would just heal itself slowly but as we approached Christmas I noticed it actually started to get worse. I am sure I overdid it on Christmas Eve and Christmas day, but I was not ready for what I would wake up to on the day after Christmas. When I went into the bathroom I looked at my incision to see if it had improved any. To my surprise, about four to five inches of the incision had totally opened up. I could actually see my insides. All I could think was, "Okay, this is not good. It is time to call the doctor!"

Of course, the doctor wanted to see me that day. I was very frustrated at this because my surgery had been eleven months prior. I had never heard of anything like this happening this far past surgery.

Once there and back in a room, my doctor looked closely at my incision. I could tell he was as shocked as me. He too said he had never had this happen before. I could tell he was very frustrated. *How did this hap-*

pen and why? He called the hospital to set up a surgery time. Though it wasn't an emergency surgery, it did need to be addressed soon before it opened up any more. Plus, he wanted to open it up a little more to better understand as to why it happened in the first place.

The only opening was on December 31. Great! Ironically, we never had plans on New Year's Eve but this year we actually had plans to go to a party with some friends. As we left the doctor's office, we just laughed about it all. We knew when we needed to laugh, and this was one of those times.

The next few days went by slowly for me. I just didn't want to wake up and see the incision had opened up anymore. Thank goodness, it didn't. I felt a little like a freak walking around with it opened up. I thought, *Nobody out there has a clue that my insides are showing.* It proves the point that nobody really knows what another person has been through even though they may look just fine in their clothes.

December 31 finally arrived. I actually did not give in to buying new pajamas this time. I just couldn't go there. I wanted to get in there, get everything fixed, and get out. I dreaded the thought of the drainage tubes that my doctor already told me I would need. At least, this time, he said I would only need two or three.

As I entered the surgery room and got on the operating table, I was looking forward to that nice five or six seconds that felt so good as they put me to sleep. Once on the table I had a very pleasant surprise. The operating table was heated. Right out loud I said, "Oh my goodness, this table is warm. Thank you!" The entire medical team in the operating room laughed at me. They were surprised I had never had a heated table considering all the surgeries I had been through in the past couple of years. I actually laid down, put out my arms, and said, "I'm ready for my anesthesia now!" I'm sure they all laughed at me and made a few comments after I went to sleep, but I didn't care. I was warm and felt really good as they put me to sleep.

Maybe at this point I was a little crazy after having so many surgeries or so many procedures and that was why I can joke like I did. I personally thought it was God who kept finding ways to help me see the humor or joy in each part of my journey.

The surgery took only two hours. Then I went to recovery for an hour and on to my room. The doctor came in to update me as to his findings. He opened up about ten inches of the incision and cleaned it out with antibiotic. He said all he could think was I had an internal infection that attacked the incision from the inside and caused the outside to open up. He did leave me with two drainage tubes and told me that he would not take them out too early.

So, there I was, down for a bit again, back to my healing couch. I was very impatient this time. I had things to do. I wasn't in the mood to stop and get better.

I went in every week for three weeks before he would agree to take out one of the drainage tubes. I could hardly do this round of drainage tubes. I had developed a sincere hate for them. He did take out one of them on the third post-op visit. That night, when I went home, I felt as sick as could be, like I had the flu or something.

But the next day, I felt better. I didn't associate feeling sick to the drainage tube at the time.

Then the next week, he agreed to take out the last drainage tube. I was very ready. I couldn't wait to be free of it. When he pulled it out, it took all I could do not to jump off the table and yell, "I'm free!" I managed to control myself and say thank you instead. He gave me instructions to not overdo it and sent me on my way.

That night I again became sick in the evening. This time I was so sick it was not funny. I threw up most the night. I never even left the toilet because I knew I would be right back in the bathroom. I made myself a pallet on the floor with a rug, a floor heater, and some comfy pajamas. By morning, I was absolutely exhausted. My husband had checked on me several times through the night and was exhausted himself for staying up with me some through the night. He had to go to work though, so he left me there and said he would check on me throughout the day. Soon after he left, I went to change clothes and noticed that my entire left breast was very red and blisters were all over my nipple. *What in the world?* I thought. *Did I burn myself sitting next to the heater all night? How did I possibly do that with my pajamas on?* It made no sense to me. I called my husband and told him about it. He too was confused as to why I was red and blistered. As the day went on I did not feel any better. I was concerned about the blisters on my breast. Would they infect that tissue? Infections seem to be my enemy!

Late in the afternoon, as I was checking to see if the redness and blisters had gone away, I noticed the other breast had become red and blistered. I knew something was wrong then. It couldn't have been the heater since the other breast was just now getting red and blistered. Something was wrong—very wrong. I immediately called my husband. He had me call the doctor. It was now four in the afternoon on a Friday afternoon. The doctor had me come in immediately. I think I already knew what he was thinking, but he didn't tell me. My husband met me at the doctor's office. The office was empty except for the staff, my husband, and me. Immediately, the nurse took me back and the doctor came in quickly. He looked at it and within seconds said, "You have Cellulitis!" He was very concerned that I would lose one if not both breasts. He put me on a high dosage of antibiotics and told me we would just have to wait and see if the antibiotics got to the infection in time. Otherwise, I would lose one or both breasts.

At this point, I was speechless. When the drainage tubes were pulled it caused internal infection that caused me to get so sick, and therefore, Cellulitis.

I went home thinking I had fought so hard to regain normalcy in how I looked and how I felt and all that might be taken away that quickly. Even though I was very upset, I knew it was out of my hands. It was in God's hands and I just had to wait and be patient. I had to let it go. God knew what he was doing in my life, and I just had to truly let it go. It was one of those times where I just had to be still.

Within just a day or two, I could see drastic improvement. I went back into the doctor and he was comfortable that I was healing and would not have to worry about losing either breast. It did take a while for it to totally go away and I developed a dark shadow under the first breast that was infected. It's a scar that I still have today.

Surgery Complete

Finally, I am able to say I am done with all the surgeries and my cancer journey. It took a year past the final surgery for me to feel like I had finally moved on, but I have.

Let me give you a recap of my journey from every surgery and procedure. I will list them in order below:

- D&C

- Hysterectomy (two weeks before cancer diagnosis)

- First biopsy

- Lumpectomy (followed up by eight weeks of radiation)

- Second biopsy and second lumpectomy

- Double mastectomy with tram flap reconstruction

- Exploratory surgery (due to problems from the tram surgery)

- Hernia surgery

- Corrective plastic surgery

- First nipple reconstruction procedure

- Second nipple reconstruction procedure

- Second exploratory surgery (to sew up incision opening)

Keep in mind that five of these surgeries required abdominal incisions. All this within a five year period of time!

Praise God that I am doing well. Though it was a long journey with many unplanned procedures and surgeries, I no longer worry about any relapse from it all. After many, many doctor visits over the past five years, I recently had my last six-month check-up, and I continue to be cancer-free. God is good. God is so good!

My New Normal

Psalms 139:14 says, "I praise you because I am fearfully and wonderfully made; your works are wonderful, I know that full well" (NIV).

That verse has even more meaning to me now that my God-given body has been through so much. I realize just how wonderfully made by God we truly are. Though I more than appreciate the doctors, especially my last plastic surgeon, who helped me find some form of normalcy since the onset of my cancer, it does not compare to my God-given body. I did not realize how comfortable I was in my body until I lost that. Anyone who has had a lot of surgery or has been in an accident that has left them less than normal can surely relate to this.

My new normal body was created by man and thus it has its limitations. For example, I do not have a lot of feeling from my chest to my lower stomach. That is due to the tram surgery. I knew that was part of it, but it doesn't feel like it did before. I always get in the shower with my backside to test the water temperature so I do not burn myself. Otherwise, I wouldn't know I was burned unless I saw it in the mirror. If you are a breast cancer survivor reading this, I know you can relate to what I am saying. I also can no longer get out of bed like normal. I have no stomach muscles so

I basically roll out of the bed each morning. At first that was such a challenge. My husband would have to help me until I got the hang of it. But now I roll out so fast, we both just laugh about it. I also cannot do sit-ups—darn! When I went back to working out, my trainer could not seem to understand this. It is not that I do not want to do them, even though I do not miss sit-ups, but I just cannot physically do them anymore!

I also cannot sleep on my stomach. I always slept on my stomach before, and now it is absolutely too uncomfortable. I have tried using pillows in every direction, but nothing seems to help.

Another discomfort I have is standing for a period of time. It becomes extremely uncomfortable for me. The mesh that was used to do my hernia surgeries left a very tight feeling and therefore, things such as standing for a long time makes me very uncomfortable. Holding a baby for too long if I am standing is very uncomfortable also. I have to sit down. This one is still upsetting to me as I love being a grandmother and insist that my grandchildren will be held by their grandmother!

Doing anything physical is more difficult for me as my stomach feels the strain of it so much more. Most days I feel fine in the morning, but very tired by the evening and usually uncomfortable in my abdomen. On a bad day, and I do have those every so often, I feel uncomfortable from the moment I get up. I just know it is a bad day. My husband has been great as he can tell without me saying a word if it is one of those days. This is my new normal, and I have accepted it because it has allowed me to look more normal and feel like a woman.

I do not have pity parties about it, but it would be wrong of me to not include it in my book. I want to add that it is because of these surgeries that I am still here, so I am grateful even though my new normal is not my original model—my God-given body that was fearfully and wonderfully made!

I considered myself very blessed from day one of learning of my cancer. God immediately gave me the verse, "Consider it pure joy my brothers, whenever you face trials of many kinds, because you know that the testing of your faith develops perseverance" (James 1:2-3 NIV), especially, the first part of the verse—consider it pure joy! I knew God would give me joy throughout this journey of my life. I knew I would have to look for the joy sometimes, but God would meet me where the joy was found. I learned God has a great sense of humor as he teaches us, specifically me. I just knew to trust and cling to that verse on the easy days and, more importantly, on the difficult ones.

In Philippians 4:7 (NIV) we are told that "the peace of God, which transcends all understanding, will guard our hearts and our minds in Jesus Christ." I lived that verse for the past five years also. Not because of anything I did or am, but because of the gracious Lord I serve. He took away any fear I should've had. I never worried, nor did I lose a moment's rest. I slept like a baby. I felt like God carried me through each surgery and procedure. I just felt *his* peace every step of the way. Truly, I had *no* fear. I always knew God was with me; whether he chose to heal me or take me home. I just had great and total peace.

I learned a lot throughout this journey. It took five years of my life from the initial diagnosis of my cancer to the healing of my last surgery. I am now a seven-year, two-time survivor of this disease. I have fought my battle but only with the help of my loving savior and Lord. He gave me one verse that I clung to throughout the entire journey and a husband and children who knew when to laugh, cry, or just listen. He also gave me a peace throughout the entire journey so I could consider it pure joy.

Two years and three months past my last surgery, I started having an unusual amount of pain on my right side. I had started working out more regularly, so I wrote it off to pulled muscles that had not been used in a long time. Unfortunately, the pain did not go away.

I was getting ready to go to my primary doctor for an annual check-up so I thought it would be wise to ask my doctor what he thought. I still was concerned about it being related to my cancer or previous treatments or surgeries in any way.

When the day of my doctor appointment arrived, I was actually anxious to hear what he thought. He immediately thought it might be a new hernia on my right side so he ordered a cat scan. As always, it was another ten days before I could get in for the scan. So once again, I was in waiting mode. I was told to schedule a follow-up doctor appointment with my plastic surgeon whom did all my corrective surgeries after the scan. My primary doctor thought maybe my plastic surgeon could check to see if this pain was related to the most recent surgery which he had done. Again, I had to wait another two weeks. My husband even took my scan to his office early so he could look at the results and let me know by phone. No call came those two weeks. Finally, the day for that appointment arrived and I was more than ready to figure out what I was dealing with and get it taken care of.

When I walked in the inner room of the doctor's office after they called my name, the doctor came in almost immediately. He had not had a chance to look at the scan, but he almost laughed at me and said, "I already know what is the matter with you. Can you not tell?"

In that moment, I was totally confused. What is he talking about? "What about that large bulge right under your chest?" he said. Yes, there was a large bulge but I just thought it was fat so I said, "I just thought I was getting fatter!" He actually laughed at my response. You might have a fluid infection there, but that is causing things to shift and subsequently causing the pain to your hip." I would never have guessed that the problem was from another area of concern, but it was.

Of course, I knew the answer to the next question. "How do I get rid of it?" Of course, he would have to go in the old incision one more time to get to it. Really? I thought those days were gone.

I was pretty much past my surgery days, so I had to really let this settle in. I couldn't believe I was scheduling another surgery. And of course I had a two week wait to get into surgery.

Actually those two weeks were great because we were in the middle of re-doing our floors downstairs and I needed the time to get my house back in order. I also wanted to have my carpets cleaned, because if I was going to be limited to my recovery couch, I needed everything to be in order so I wouldn't be tempted to get up and clean.

The morning of the surgery arrived, and it was the same routine as always. But this time, I would be at a different hospital that my doctor likes to do his surgeries at. It was a newer facility and very nice. The staff was wonderful and one step ahead of me, which is funny since I brag on knowing this routine so well. The nurse came in and gave me my lovely gown and hospital socks. Though I brought my own socks, I decided to be a good patient and just wear the ones provided. My husband and children came up and entertained me to make the time go by. It actually went by very fast. The anesthesiologist came in and talked to me. He actually laughed a little when he looked at my chart and noticed how many surgeries I have had. He knew I knew the routine, so his visit was brief. Then my plastic surgeon came in and asked everyone to leave so he could draw on me for my surgery. He brought two interns with him that I had never met before. Though I am a private person I decided to say nothing as they stayed for him to discuss with me each part of the surgery as he drew on my abdomen.

After he left, my husband and children prayed over me. I was calm and felt ready to take surgery on one more time. The nurse came in with a shot that she said would start to make me weary and I probably wouldn't remember much after that. I remember looking at my family as if to say "No, I still feel normal," but that is the last thing I remember until I was on the operating table, and I felt them putting on some compressive stockings.

The next thing I knew, I was in recovery. I woke up to a very bad sore throat. I also had to go to the bathroom really badly. I told the nurse I needed to get up and go so she went to help me. As I sat up, instead of one nurse, I saw three, and there were blue stars all around. The next thing I knew, I was lying almost off the bed and there were several nurses around me. "You left us for a bit honey!" She told me she could not let me get out of bed, so I would have to use a bed pan. I doubted I could, but I decided give it a shot. She put it underneath me and then proceeded to stay in the room. She just stood there waiting. I told her I could not go with her in the room, so she left. Unfortunately, I could not go when she left the room either. Plain and simple, I just could not pee while I was lying down.

She then let my husband and children back to see me. We talked for a few minutes and again, I asked to go to the bathroom. She decided to let me try and get out of bed again. I sat up, thought I was doing a little better, but down I went. I passed out again.

At this point she was not taking any more chances. She said you will have to try the bed pan again. So, she had everyone leave, put it underneath me, and then left the room. I told her I needed a few minutes. It probably took me ten minutes, but I finally was able to go.

Even though this was an outpatient surgery, they insisted I stay until eight o'clock that evening so they could make sure I was okay since I had passed out twice. Reluctantly, I said okay, but I was not happy about it. My family was there to keep me laughing so the day did pass by pretty quickly. Finally, at seven that evening, they said I was released to leave. We quickly packed up our belongings and were on our way home.

I didn't enjoy the ride home, as I never did, because every bump seemed worse when I had abdominal surgery. I just held my gut the whole way home and headed for my couch. I knew a nap would surely help, and it did.

I was tougher this surgery. I made myself sleep in my bed from the first night home. It is hard to get up in our bed, but I insisted. I also took very little medicine from the first day home. I allowed myself to take a muscle relaxer sometimes during the day and just one pain reliever at bedtime so I could get to sleep. I knew in the long run this would be a wise idea. No regrets.

The weekend went by quickly, and my biggest complaint was probably just being tired. The pain was definitely manageable.

The best part of it all was I no longer had pain in my side and the large bulge under my chest was gone. That was just awesome! I may have had surgery pain, but I felt so much better. The surgery definitely solved my problem.

On Monday, three days later, I went to the doctor's office for my post-op appointment. I didn't get to talk to the doctor after surgery, so I was looking forward to hearing what he had to say. My husband took me as I could not yet drive. When the doctor walked in, he could tell by the look on my face that I was feeling pretty good. He proceeded to tell me that there was no infection at all (that is really great news). He went on to tell me that a large piece of tissue had literally died and was very, very hard. He said it was also quite challenging to get out. He believed it formed after the last surgery two years ago, and slowly, the cells died off, leaving it very hard and uncomfortable. It was putting pressure on other organs causing the pain in my side. It appeared to me that it was a very necessary surgery. I am glad I addressed it. He wasn't comfortable taking out my drainage tube just yet. He suggested ordering a special body girdle so as to not allow tissue to do that this time. So, of course, I ordered it.

I am determined to follow every order completely because I would love to be done with surgery at this point. While a friend was visiting during the week after surgery, she asked how many surgeries I have had related to my cancer journey. "This surgery will make 13!" I said.

"Really," said my oldest, "That makes a baker's dozen!" I think it's absolutely wonderful that my own children carry the gene to find humor and joy in any situation.

This surgery went very well to say the least. Family and friends visited, brought food and flowers, and prayed with me. My last drainage tube came out ten days after surgery, and I am healing more each day.

I learned a new lesson this time. My journey continues. Even if I get cancer back in my life again, need another treatment, procedure, or surgery, or remain cancer-free, it is part of my life journey. God continues to give me peace, great rest, and an incredible amount of joy every single day.

I have also learned to embrace the entire verse:

> Consider it pure joy, my brothers, whenever you
> face trials of many kinds, because you know that
> the testing of your faith develops perseverance.
>
> James 1:2-3

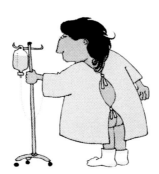